TEST MODULE

for NCLEX-RN
Questions/Answers/Rationales

STAFF

Clinical Editor
Marguerite Ambrose, RN,CS, MSN, CCRN

Clinical Reviewer
Judith E. Meissner, RN, MSN

Copy Editor
Jane Benner

Cover Design
Jake Smith

CONTRIBUTORS

Nursing Fundamentals
Kathleen M. Maher, RN, MSN

Mental Health Nursing
Carol Bininger, RN, PhD
Gail Iglesias, RN, EdD

Pediatric Nursing
Nancy Wallace, RN,C, MSN

Medical/Surgical Nursing
Kay Scharn, RN, MSN, EdS

Maternity Nursing
S. Kim Genovese, RNC, MSN, MSA

Pharmacology
James Lile, PharmD

CONTENTS

Ace It! Test Module

CHAPTER 1

Introduction

TEST MODULE

Introduction

The *Ace It!* Test Module is an important part of your study program for the NCLEX-RN. It contains more than 500 questions divided into two integrated tests and four tests within clinical areas. Knowing how to accurately analyze test questions, learning strategies for successful test-taking, and building self-confidence that you can answer NCLEX-RN questions are crucial to passing the exam. The *Ace It!* Test Module is designed to help you achieve these goals. To maximize your benefit from this module, you should use it in conjunction with the *Ace It!* Study Guide Module.

Understanding the NCLEX-RN

The NCLEX-RN is a computerized exam in which questions of varying levels of difficulty are presented to you on a computer. You will be required to answer enough questions correctly to demonstrate your competence as a beginning practitioner.

The NCLEX-RN is a computer adaptive test (CAT). This means that the test adapts the difficulty of a question to the response you gave to the previous question. For example, if you answer a question incorrectly, the next question will be easier. If you answer a question correctly, the next question will be more difficult. Since the computer adapts its question selection to your response, the exam is individualized for you.

The NCLEX-RN test bank contains thousands of questions, categorized by level of difficulty, clinical area, and client need. The process of giving you questions based on your response to the previous question continues until the computer can determine that you have demonstrated competence in all areas of the NCLEX-RN test plan.

When you begin your exam, you will get some instructions on how to use the computer and will be given a short practice session. One question at a time will appear on the computer screen; some will have a short clinical situation presented and others will be stand-alone questions. All questions will have four possible answers.

Everyone will get at least 75 questions. After answering 75 questions, you may find that your exam ends; that means that the computer has sufficient information to conclude that you are or are not going to pass the test. On the other hand, if the computer cannot yet determine whether you will pass the test, it will continue giving you questions (up to 265 over a 5-hour period).

The test will end when the computer has determined your competence. You will not be given a score at the test center. Results of your test will be mailed to you, usually within a few weeks. In some states, you can telephone the Board of Nursing to get your results.

One of the *Ace It!* modules is an actual computerized test (CAT) just like the real NCLEX-RN. You will be instructed in the Study Guide Module when to use it.

The NCLEX-RN test plan
The NCLEX-RN is based on a test plan that organizes questions according to client need categories that define all nursing actions and competencies across all health care settings for all clients. There are four main categories and 10 subcategories. Each category has a predetermined number of questions based on a job analysis of nursing duties of entry-level registered nurses. The test plan categories, a brief description of each, and the percentage of questions assigned to each are listed below.

NCLEX-RN test categories
Category and percentage of questions
A. Safe, effective care environment
   1. Management of care--7% to 13% (providing coordinated, integrated, cost-effective care, supervising and collaborating with other health team members)
   2. Safety and infection control--5% to 11% (protecting clients and staff from health hazards)
B. Health promotion and maintenance
   3. Growth & development through the life span--7% to 13% (assisting client and family through normal stages of development from birth through old age)
   4. Prevention and early detection of disease--5% to 11% (providing and managing care for the prevention and and early detection of disease)
C. Psychosocial integrity
   5. Coping and adaptation--5% to 11% (promoting the client's ability to cope and adapt to illness or stressful events)
   6. Psychosocial adaptation--5% to 11% (managing and providing care for clients with mental illness)

D. Physiological integrity
    7. Basic care and comfort--7% to 13% (providing comfort and assistance in activities of daily living)
    8. Pharmacologic and parenteral therapies--5% to 11% (managing and administering drugs and parenteral therapies)
    9. Reduction of risk potential--12% to 18% (reducing the likelihood of complications or health problems developing)
    10. Physiological adaptation--12% to 18% (managing and providing care for acute, chronic, or life-threatening health conditions)

Integrated throughout the exam are the concepts of: Nursing process; Caring; Communication; Cultural awareness; Documentation; Self-care; Teaching/Learning. These concepts are fundamental to the practice of professional nursing and testing of them will be found in all the client need categories. A more detailed explanation of the new NCLEX-RN can be found on the *Ace It!* Video Module.

Successful hints for taking the NCLEX-RN
Mastering the ability to pass an examination is based on thoroughly studying the subject and applying well-proven strategies of successful test-taking. These 20 hints can dramatically improve your chances of success on NCLEX-RN. Read and remember them.

- **TEST-TAKING HINT #1:** Remember that "why" questions can often put a client on the defensive, so a nurse's response that begins with "why" is most likely not the correct answer to a question. Keep this hint in mind as you analyze questions.

- **TEST-TAKING HINT #2:** Try answering the questions without looking at the answers (put your hand over the answers on the computer screen). Then look at the answer choices. If the answer you selected is among the choices, it most likely is the correct one. This technique is a good test of your critical thinking skills.

- **TEST-TAKING HINT #3:** Read each case study carefully. It has all the data you need to answer the question correctly. Do not read information into the case or the question. Each case and question stand alone; they do not rely on data from previous cases or questions.

- **TEST-TAKING HINT #4:** Remember that NCLEX questions usually require a high level of discrimination. Look carefully for words like *best, first, most, highest priority*. All the answer options may be plausible but only one will meet the discriminator.

- **TEST-TAKING HINT #5:** Read *all* answer options carefully before making your selection and again before confirming your selection (the computerized NCLEX requires you to confirm the answer selection you have made, but once you have confirmed your choice, you cannot go back and change it). This will prevent one of the main causes of wrong answers, failing to read the question and *all* options carefully.

- **TEST-TAKING HINT #6:** Don't cram for the NCLEX. You already have enough facts. Practice making sure you can apply what you know. Remember, you have done well enough to get to this point, so there's no reason you shouldn't succeed on the exam.

- **TEST-TAKING HINT #7:** Know what the question really is asking. Analyze the stem and the actual question, which may not always end with a question mark. For example:

  > A child receiving chemotherapy for leukemia is
  > encouraged to play. You understand that play
  > activity's goal is to
  > 1. help the child to communicate.
  > 2. let him express anger over his illness.
  > 3. assess the child's knowledge of the disease process.
  > 4. build the child's spirits.
  > Correct answer - 1
  > The question is asking what is the play activity
  > goal? Only number 1 is a goal of play. The
  > others are distractors.

- **TEST-TAKING HINT #8:** Know your weak areas. You probably knew which clinical areas and client need categories you were most unsure of before you started reviewing, and the pre-test likely confirmed this. Keep those weak areas in mind as you progress through *Ace It!*. After the post-test, analyze the results to see what progress you made.

- **TEST-TAKING HINT #9:** If you're not sure which answer option to choose, try grouping the answers using common sense. This will usually leave you with two likely choices. Analyze each of them using your critical thinking skills and select the one that makes the most sense to you. You probably are right.

- **TEST-TAKING HINT #10:** When asked to select the *best* nurse's response to a client's question or comment, eliminate any answer option that offers false reassurance, such as "Everything is going to be alright." You may not have enough data to say that, so it is probably a wrong choice. See the therapeutic communications section of the review book.

- **TEST-TAKING HINT #11:** When a question is asking you about a drug, remember the "5 rights of medication administration": Right client, right drug, right route, right dose, right time. You also may want to consider allergy history and expiration date of drug. This will help you as you analyze the answer options.

- **TEST-TAKING HINT #12:** Don't select an answer option that states, "Call the health care provider," unless you are sure there is no appropriate nursing action you should take *first*. Calling the health care provider may be appropriate, but other options that make you to do something for the client probably have priority.

- **TEST-TAKING HINT #13:** Client safety is a nursing priority, and assuring this takes precedence over all other actions. Client safety questions are 15% to 21% of all questions asked on the NCLEX.

- **TEST-TAKING HINT #14:** Remember that maintaining a patent airway has the highest priority. It is always the correct choice when asked what is "first," "most important," or "best" nursing action to take when dealing with a client with an airway problem.

- **TEST-TAKING HINT #15:** Know what you must *teach* a client when a drug is prescribed. Teaching should include adverse effects, dosage schedule, taking the drug on empty or full stomach, completing full treatment regimen, and--most important-- not to discontinue drugs abruptly.

- **TEST-TAKING HINT #16:** Know the major adverse effects, important nursing implications, and client teaching to give for commonly prescribed drugs. These can be grouped according to drug category. For example, diuretics deplete potassium levels. Because they cause the body to lose water, intake and output and weight are important nursing considerations during diuretic therapy. Remember, you are not going to see questions on NCLEX about drugs that are rarely prescribed or used only in highly specialized care units.

- **TEST-TAKING HINT #17:** Trust that there are no trick questions on NCLEX. The exam's sole purpose is to evaluate your ability to be a safe practitioner and to be sure that you can apply nursing concepts and principles safely.

- **TEST-TAKING HINT #18:** Prepare yourself, physically and emotionally, a few days before the examination.
    1. Know how to get to the site and how long it takes to get there. Try to

arrive 5 or 10 minutes early so you can get comfortable with the testing center.
2. Be sure to get a good night's sleep. Try to take the day before the test off from work.
3. Eat moderately. A bloated feeling doesn't help with concentration.
4. Wear clothing you can add or shed depending on test-center temperatures.

- **TEST-TAKING HINT #19:** Learn a relaxation exercise that you know works for you--maybe just taking a deep breath or using imagery. Use the exercise if you find yourself getting uptight. Remember, the average test-taker completes the exam in 90 minutes.

- **TEST-TAKING HINT #20:** Finally, remember all you've learned here. Review your weak areas. Build a positive attitude. Tell yourself that you are a good nurse and are going to be successful on NCLEX-RN.

Taking the tests
Ace It! **Pre-test**
The *Ace It!* Pre-test evaluates your knowledge base of nursing prior to beginning your review for the NCLEX-RN. By completing the diagnostic profile at the end of the test and analyzing the results, you will have a good idea of any test-taking weaknesses and nursing areas that will need concentrated study to assure your readiness for NCLEX-RN.

The pre-test consists of 70 questions, covering all clinical nursing areas and all areas of the NCLEX-RN test plan. All pre-test questions are at the same or higher level of difficulty as on the actual exam.

When you take the pre-test, pay attention to the time it took you to finish. The actual NCLEX-RN does not assign a specific amount of time for answering each question, but there is a maximum of 5 hours permitted to complete the exam. If you take more than 90 minutes to complete the pre-test, you may want to make a note to remind yourself that you will have to speed up answering questions so you do not run out of total time.

After completing the test, score it using the answer key at the end of the test. Complete the diagnostic profile and use its results to focus your study plan.

Clinical tests
There are four clinical tests covering Mental Health Nursing, Pediatric Nursing, Medical/Surgical Nursing, and Maternity Nursing. Each test has a sufficient number of questions to evaluate your knowledge base in each area. Follow the Study Guide Module for when to take the clinical area tests.

To help you evaluate your ability to answer correctly questions covering all client need categories, each question is coded for the appropriate client need category. All client need categories covered by the NCLEX-RN are included in the clinical area test questions.

The clinical tests are organized with the question in the left column and the answer in the right column. Use an index card to cover the right-hand column until you have selected your answer to the question. Then lower the card to reveal the answer. Mark whether you answered it correctly or incorrectly. Having the answer across from the question eliminates your having to continually flip back and forth from the front to the back of the book as in many Q & A books.

As in the *Ace It!* Pre-test, use the diagnostic profile at the end of each test to analyze your performance. You will have a graphic picture of whether you need further study in any clinical area or client need category.

Ace It! **Post-test**
The *Ace It!* Post-test is the final step in your study program for the NCLEX-RN. The *Ace It!* Study Guide Module will instruct you when to begin this test.

The *Ace It!* Post-test consists of 90 items, covering all clinical areas and all areas of the NCLEX-RN Test Plan. Each question is written in the same format as those on the actual NCLEX-RN.

Mark the option you select by circling it. After you complete the *Ace It!* Post-test, check your answer selections against the answer key at the end of the test. Each question is coded two ways: Clinical Area and Client Need Category. Calculate your subscores for these two categories using the tables following the answer key.

Because the post-test is not a mirror of the actual NCLEX-RN Test Plan, it is not a predictor of your performance on the real exam. However, it a good indicator of your readiness. A score under 75 would indicate your need for another review of the *Ace It!* content and a need for a more in-depth study of specific nursing areas.

CHAPTER 2

Ace It! Pre-test

Instructions

This pretest consists of 70 individual questions. Each question is followed by four possible answers. Read each question and all possible answers carefully, then select the best answer. Remember, *each question has only one correct answer*. Circle the answer you have selected.

Answer each question as it is presented before you move on to the next question. The computerized exam will not allow you to pass a question without answering it.

After you have completed the test, check your responses against the correct answers provided in the "Answer Key with Rationale" section that immediately follows this test. The major purpose of comparing your answers to the test items and the key is to provide further guidance for studying before NCLEX-RN. Each question in the pretest is coded by category of client need (CN) and clinical area (CA). The codes follow the rationales.

For the items you answered correctly, review the rationales to make sure that you got the right answer for the right *reason*. Review the items you answered incorrectly. Was it because you didn't know the content or was it because you marked an answer incorrectly by mistake?

After you have looked at each of the rationales complete the Personal Diagnostic Profile and calculate the subscores as explained immediately following the Answer Key with Rationale. Evaluate your overall performance on the test. If you got scores below 75% in a category, focus on that area during your review process.

1. A 3-year-old girl is being observed for symptoms of sickle-cell anemia, which include
   1. beefy, red tongue.
   2. painful joints.
   3. urinary retention.
   4. carpopedal spasms.

2. The nurse observes a female client for symptoms of anorexia nervosa, which include
   1. tachycardia.
   2. increased blood pressure.
   3. decreased physical activity.
   4. amenorrhea.

3. A client has had a cardiac catheterization that was performed percutaneously through the femoral artery. Which of these measures should be included in the client's care following the procedure?
   1. Restricting oral fluids for 8 hours.
   2. Observing the puncture site for bleeding frequently.
   3. Maintaining a high-Fowler's position for several hours.
   4. Performing passive exercises to the affected extremity every hour.

4. A client is given instructions to avoid foods that are high in potassium. He shows that he has understood the instructions if he selects which of these foods as *highest* in potassium?
   1. One slice of toasted, white bread.
   2. One large, boiled egg.
   3. One medium banana.
   4. One cup of corn flakes.

5. The nurse teaches a primigravida about what to expect during pregnancy. The client shows that she understands what she was taught if she states that she expects to first feel quickening at which of these weeks of gestation?
   1. 8 to 11   3. 16 to 22
   2. 12 to 15   4. 23 to 29

6. A 21-year-old primigravida arrives at the clinic because she suspects she is pregnant. Which statement reveals that she has a common symptom seen early in pregnancy?
   1. "My breasts feel so full."
   2. "I have tingling sensations in my fingertips."
   3. "After I brush my hair there is lots of hair in the brush."
   4. "I seem to have extra bursts of energy."

7. A client complains of fatigue, anorexia, abdominal pain, and generalized weakness. He also has a cardiac arrhythmia and decreased reflexes. Given this information, the nurse should suspect that he has which of these electrolyte imbalances?
   1. Hypokalemia   3. Hypocalcemia
   2. Hypernatremia   4. Hypermagnesemia

8. Which of the following neuroleptic drugs would the nurse expect to see prescribed for a 70-year-old client with acute psychosis?
   1. Mellaril (thioridazine)
   2. Haldol (haloperidol)
   3. Sinequan (doxepin)
   4. Noctec (chloral hydrate)

9. A client is to get an I.V. infusion of 3,000 ml of 5% dextrose in water over a 24-hour period. The drip factor on the infusion delivers 15 drops/ml. The client's infusion should be set to deliver about how many drops per minute?
   1. 10   3. 30
   2. 20   4. 40

10. A client has just been told that a tumor removed from her lung is cancerous. She begins sobbing uncontrollably. Which action should the nurse take?
    1. Remain with the client and let her cry.
    2. Leave the room and find out if the client can have a sedative.
    3. Ask the client exactly what her health care provider told her.
    4. Explain that it is important for the client not to cry now.

11. A client who has had abdominal surgery is complaining of pain and has abdominal distention. Which of these measures should be included in her care plan?
    1. Give the client ice chips to suck on.
    2. Listen for the client's bowel sounds.
    3. Encourage the client to remain in a side-lying position.
    4. Apply a binder to the client's abdomen.

12. The presence of an esophageal atresia with a tracheoesophageal fistula should be considered in a newborn who has which one of these symptoms?
    1. Ineffective sucking
    2. Projectile vomiting
    3. Sternal retractions
    4. Choking

13. A client with long-term schizophrenia claims to be getting messages from the CIA through the television. Antipsychotic medication is prescribed. Which one of these statements made by the client indicates that the medication was effective?
    1. "The CIA messages are coming through the radio now instead of the television."
    2. "The CIA messages aren't coming as often now."
    3. "I take my medication every day, even though I don't want to."
    4. "I get a little dizzy when I get up from a chair."

14. A 40-year-old client, newly diagnosed with lung cancer that has metastasized to the bone, says to the nurse, "I can't believe that this cancer is so advanced. I didn't have symptoms until very recently." The nurse's response should be based on which of these understandings about lung cancer?
    1. Chemotherapeutic agents have made the cure rate for metastatic lung cancer excellent.
    2. The younger the client is when the diagnosis of lung cancer is made, the better his chances of survival.
    3. In many cases, symptoms of lung cancer first appear when the disease is far advanced.
    4. The threshold for pain generally is elevated in clients who do not notice early symptoms of lung cancer.

15. A pregnant client explains that she does not eat red meat or eggs, but does include milk and cheese in her diet. Her plan of care *must* include a supplemental source of which one of these nutrients?
    1. Calcium.
    2. Iron.
    3. Carotene (vitamin A).
    4. Ascorbic acid (vitamin C).

16. A client is admitted to the hospital because of a cerebrovascular accident (CVA). She is non-responsive. When doing a neurological check, the nurse notices that the client's pupils respond very slowly to light. Which of these questions should the nurse consider *initially?*
    1. Does the client have other symptoms of meningitis?
    2. What other signs of an impending seizure are present?
    3. Does the client have other signs of increased intracranial pressure?
    4. What other symptoms of pressure on the hypothalamus are present?

17. When a child is getting cyclophosphamide (Cytoxan), the results of which one of these blood tests is *most* important for the nurse to monitor?
    1. Prothrombin time
    2. Leukocyte count
    3. Urea nitrogen
    4. Total bilirubin

18. A client is admitted to the hospital because of acute pancreatitis. The nurse gets all of the following data about the client. Which one is *most* likely related to the development of his pancreatitis?
    1. He has had a hiatal hernia for 15 years.
    2. He has abused alcohol for 10 years.
    3. He had a sore throat about 6 months ago.
    4. He has been taking antacids for about three months.

19. A client develops left ventricular dysfunction secondary to an MI. During the physical assessment, the nurse would expect to find
    1. bilateral basilar crackles.
    2. elevated central venous pressure.
    3. pitting sacral edema.
    4. hepatojugular reflex.

20. An elderly client has had a transurethral prostatectomy for benign prostatic hyperplasia. The client has received discharge instructions. Which one of these statements made by the client indicates that he understood the instruction?
    1. "Eating a bland, low-residue diet is best until my urethra is completely healed."
    2. "For the next few weeks, I will probably continue to have some burning when I urinate."
    3. "I am best off sitting instead of walking or lying down."
    4. "I will need to make an appointment to have the stitches removed."

21. A primigravida who is 10 weeks pregnant calls the nurse at the clinic to report that she is experiencing slight vaginal bleeding and pelvic cramps. Which of these instructions by the nurse is *most* appropriate at this time?
    1. "Save any perineal pads, clots, or tissue and come to the clinic right away."
    2. "Lie down on your left side and call again if the flow increases."
    3. "Avoid exercise and sexual intercourse for the next 2 weeks."
    4. "Continue your normal activities and increase your fluid intake."

22. A 2½-year-old child is admitted to the hospital in cardiac failure. The nurse should assess him for which of these symptoms associated with cardiac failure?
    1. Low-grade fever
    2. Dyspnea
    3. Weight loss
    4. Bounding pulse

23. A nurses' aide is assigned to care for an elderly client who has a hearing impairment affecting both ears. To facilitate communication with this client, the nurse should instruct the aide to take which of these measures?
    1. "Use a high-pitched tone of voice when speaking to this client."
    2. "Speak directly into this client's ear."
    3. "Stand with your face at this client's eye level before speaking."
    4. "Maintain a distance of about 8 feet from this client when speaking to her."

24. A 4-year-old child is being treated with digoxin (Lanoxin) for heart failure. The child should be observed for adverse effects of Lanoxin, which include
    1. a loss of appetite.
    2. a urine specific gravity of 1.010.
    3. euphoria.
    4. yellowish sclera.

25. An 8-month-old baby girl is being observed
    for symptoms of bronchiolitis, which include
    1. diarrhea and swollen lymph glands.
    2. fever and cough.
    3. sore throat and Koplik's spots.
    4. facial rash and vomiting.

26. A client in the 39th week of pregnancy is
    admitted to the hospital in active labor. The
    nurse takes the fetal heart rate and finds it to
    be 80 beats per minute. Which action should
    the nurse take *next?*
    1. Record the fetal heart rate findings.
    2. Place the client in shock position.
    3. Check the mother's pulse rate.
    4. Encourage the client to take deep breaths.

27. A nurse is teaching a client about the
    procedure for obtaining a clean-catch urine
    specimen. The nurse's instructions should
    include which of these statements?
    1. "Don't eat or drink anything for 6 hours
       before the procedure."
    2. "Use a clean, rather than sterile, container
       to collect the urine."
    3. "Cleanse your perineum using a motion
       that moves from the back to the front."
    4. "Start urinating, stop, then urinate into the
       collection container."

28. A client in the second trimester of pregnancy
    confides to the nurse that she has been
    smoking a pack of cigarettes a day. She states,
    "I'm afraid to deliver a big baby, and I've
    heard that smoking results in smaller babies."
    Which of these responses, by the nurse, is
    appropriate?
    1. "Smoking is not the best way to ensure a
       small baby. Instead, you should limit your
       dietary intake to 1,200 calories or less a
       day."
    2. "A small baby has a higher risk of
       developmental problems at birth. Let's talk
       about smoking."
    3. "That is just not true. Your baby's size is

determined by multiple factors unrelated to
smoking."
    4. "I can understand your concern. Smoking a
       few cigarettes a day should not harm the
       baby."

29. A newborn is born with a myelomeningocele
    at the second lumbar vertebra. Because of the
    defect, it would be *essential* for the nurse to
    observe the infant frequently for presence of
    1. infection.
    2. hemorrhage.
    3. bilirubinemia.
    4. hyperkalemia.

30. A female client is admitted to the hospital
    because it is suspected that she has Addison's
    disease. Symptoms of Addison's disease
    include
    1. increase in facial hair.
    2. skin that bruises easily.
    3. hyperglycemia.
    4. hypotension.

31. A client who had abdominal surgery 2 days
    earlier has developed a thrombophlebitis in his
    right leg. Which of these notations should be
    made on his care plan?
    1. "Keep right leg below the level of the
       heart."
    2. "Discourage the client from staying in
       bed."
    3. "Avoid rubbing the right leg."
    4. "Apply moist, cold packs to the right leg.

32. A nurse is orienting a new practical nurse about the care of a client who is to have a temporary sealed source of internal radiation therapy (cesium) for cervical cancer. The nurse should give the practical nurse which of these instructions about the client's care after the implantation of the radiation?
    1. "Make sure that an aluminum-lined container with long forceps is in the room at all times in case the radiation source becomes dislodged."
    2. "Check the client's soiled linen to make sure that the source of radiation has not fallen out."
    3. "To minimize exposure to the radiation, pregnant staff members should plan to complete their direct care activities for the client in 30 minutes."
    4. "Encourage the client to walk around as much as possible to prevent complications from the radiation."

33. During the acute phase of alcohol detoxification, which one of these measures should be included in the client's plan of care?
    1. Maintain seizure precautions.
    2. Keep the client's room brightly lit.
    3. Restrict the client's fluids to 1,000 ml per day.
    4. Apply wrist and ankle restraints.

34. Which activity will best meet the growth and development needs of an 8-year-old girl?
    1. Giving her blocks to play with.
    2. Encouraging her to watch television.
    3. Playing a board game with a child her age.
    4. Having her mother read a schoolbook to her.

35. A client who has increased intracranial pressure from a head injury is to get I.V. mannitol (Osmitrol). It is prescribed for which of these purposes?
    1. To restore electrolytes.
    2. To stimulate kidney function.
    3. To increase circulating blood volume.
    4. To reduce cerebral edema.

36. A client with acquired immunodeficiency syndrome (AIDS) is admitted to hospital with *Pneumocystis carinii* pneumonia (PCP). On admission, he can be expected to have which of these notations in the care plan?
    1. "Offer frequent oral hygiene."
    2. "Add a small amount of hydrogen peroxide to bath water."
    3. "Administer a stool softener."
    4. "Restrict intake of high-protein foods."

37. A 3-year-old boy is admitted to the hospital with nephrotic syndrome. His care plan should include which of these statements?
    1. "Test urine for acetone."
    2. "Encourage fluid intake."
    3. "Keep room cool."
    4. "Provide meticulous skin care."

38. A client is hospitalized because he sustained an incomplete transection of the spinal cord at the first and second lumbar vertebrae as a result of an accident. Since the injury, he has been unable to move his lower extremities. His wife asks the nurse if her husband will ever be able to walk again. The nurse's response should be based on which of these understandings about the husband's potential for rehabilitation?
    1. His deficits are permanent because the initial trauma to the spinal cord is irreparable.
    2. His deficits are permanent because motor nerves in the spinal cord have been traumatized.
    3. His deficits cannot be accurately determined until spinal shock to the spinal cord subsides.
    4. His deficits cannot be accurately determined until replacement of the motor nerves in the spinal cord is complete.

39. A nurse is helping evaluate the care plan of a client who has been admitted to the hospital in severe pain resulting from a calculus in his right kidney. Because the client is in the acute stage of his illness, the nurse should expect that which of these measures is being included in his care plan?
    1. Keeping cold compresses on his right flank area.
    2. Instructing him to lie on his right side when he is in bed.
    3. Restricting fluid intake to 1,000 ml a day.
    4. Straining his urine through gauze after each voiding.

40. A client who has severe chest pain is admitted to the hospital with a myocardial infarction. After evaluating the client, a health care provider writes all of the following orders. Which one should the nurse *question?*
    1. Morphine sulfate 15 mg q4h I.M. prn.
    2. Oxygen via nasal cannula at 4 liters/minute prn.
    3. Full liquid diet as tolerated.
    4. Colace 50 mg b.i.d.

41. After a normal newborn infant is bottle fed, the nurse should place the infant in which of these positions?
    1. Supine, with his head slightly elevated.
    2. Prone, with his head slightly lowered.
    3. Left-side lying.
    4. Right-side lying.

42. A 10-year-old boy with a history of sickle-cell anemia is admitted to the hospital in vasoocclusive (thrombocytic) crisis. The nurse should give *priority* to which one of these nursing diagnoses in the child's care plan?
    1. Pain related to tissue ischemia.
    2. Anxiety related to hospitalization.
    3. Fatigue related to anemia.
    4. Knowledge deficit related to prevention of crisis.

43. A client who is hospitalized because of severe bacterial pneumonia is having difficulty coughing up thick, tenacious sputum. In planning measures to help loosen his respiratory secretions, the nurse should definitely collect data about
    1. the client's fluid intake.
    2. the client's tidal volume.
    3. whether the client is breathing through pursed lips.
    4. whether the client is placed in Trendelenburg position periodically.

44. A nurse works at a women's health center where many of the clients are recent immigrants from Southeast Asian countries. Because of the clients' cultural norms, the nurse should expect to observe which of these behaviors?
    1. They prefer to be treated by male rather than female care-givers.
    2. They avoid eye contact when speaking to the staff.
    3. They seek advice from health professionals rather than their family.
    4. They report mental symptoms more readily than physical symptoms.

45. A client in labor is having contractions every 3 minutes, lasting 45 to 60 seconds. Examination reveals that her cervix is 100% effaced and dilated 6 cm. Based on this information, the nurse should identify that the client is in which of these phases of labor?
    1. Latent
    2. Active
    3. Transitional
    4. End of first stage

46. Which nursing measure should be included in the care plan of a client with chronic renal failure?
    1. Observing him for signs of dehydration.
    2. Monitoring him for increased hemoglobin levels.
    3. Providing him with a diet high in protein.
    4. Weighing him each day.

47. A child is admitted to the hospital because of acute bacterial meningitis. The child is placed on universal precautions. In addition, the child should be placed on which of these types of isolation for about 24 to 48 hours after the start of antibiotic therapy?
    1. Enteric
    2. Protective
    3. Respiratory
    4. Wound and skin

48. A client's husband died 10 months ago after a brief illness. To help her cope with her loss, she has participated as a member of a bereavement group for the last 6 months. Which statement indicates that the client is reaching resolution of the grieving process?
    1. "I plan to get out and do some volunteer work at the church my husband and I attended."
    2. "I hope that I will wake up from this bad dream and find my husband still alive."
    3. "I see people on the bus or in a store who I mistake for my husband."
    4. "I think if I had forced him to go to a doctor sooner, he would still be alive."

49. A female client is admitted to the hospital with a diagnosis of heart failure. Which of these findings in her history is *most* closely related to the development of this condition?
    1. She is accustomed to wearing tight-fitting undergarments.
    2. She has an elevated blood pressure.
    3. She was treated for pulmonary tuberculosis 2 years ago.
    4. She worked as a waitress until her retirement 3 years ago.

50. A 3-month-old male infant who had a developmental dysplasia of his right hip has had a Frejka pillow splint applied. Which of these findings indicates that the procedure has corrected the infant's defect?
    1. The infant is able to turn more easily from side to side.
    2. The circumference of the infant's thighs are equal in size.
    3. The infant is able to fully abduct his affected extremity.
    4. The femoral pulse is palpable on the infant's affected side.

51. A client was admitted to the burn unit of a hospital for treatment of burns. The client has burns on the face, chest, and abdomen. In terms of the burns on the client's abdomen, the skin appears very red and blistered. The client complains that the area is very painful. The client's burns would be classified as
    1. first degree.
    2. second degree.
    3. third degree.
    4. fourth degree.

52. A client has just been informed that he has rectal cancer and will need to have a colostomy. He asks the nurse, "How will I ever get through this horrible operation?" Which of these responses of the nurse is appropriate?
    1. "Don't worry about the operation. You're in very good hands."
    2. "Thousands of people have this operation and do just fine."
    3. "Aren't you thankful that such an operation is available to cure you?"
    4. "What does this operation mean to you?"

53. A client was being prepared for an exploratory laparotomy. His wife was present when he was given his preoperative medications, which included meperidine (Demerol) hydrochloride. About 15 minutes after he got his preoperative medications, the nurse determines that he has not signed a consent form for the surgery. It would be *best* for the nurse to take which of these actions next?
    1. Notify the charge nurse.
    2. Have the client sign the consent form.
    3. Ask the client's wife to sign the consent form.
    4. Document the incident in the client's chart.

54. Following delivery of the placenta, a client is given methylergonovine maleate (Methergine). The nurse should observe the client for the drug's adverse effects, which include
    1. hypertension.
    2. hypoglycemia.
    3. uterine atony.
    4. urinary retention.

55. On the first day after a transurethral resection, a client complains of severe pain in his suprapubic area. He has an indwelling urethral catheter, which is attached to gravity drainage and an analgesic order. Which of these actions should the nurse take *first?*
    1. Apply the Credé maneuver to his suprapubic area.
    2. Determine when he last got an analgesic.
    3. Check the patency of his urinary catheter.
    4. Reposition him in bed.

56. A client who has grand mal seizures is to take phenytoin (Dilantin) sodium. Which one of these statements indicates that he is aware of an adverse effect of Dilantin?
    1. "The drug may make me drowsy."
    2. "The drug will make me urinate more frequently."
    3. "It is likely my hair will begin to fall out."
    4. "It is likely my weight will increase."

57. A newborn infant has an Apgar score of 4 at 2 minutes after birth, and resuscitation measures are instituted. At 5 minutes after birth, the nurse determines the Apgar score from the following data:
    - Heart rate: 130 beats per minute
    - Respiratory effort: Good, crying
    - Muscle tone: Some flexion of extremities
    - Reflex irritability: Weak cry
    - Color: Body pink, extremities blue

(Question continued on next page)

(Question number 57 continued)

Based on these data, the nurse should conclude that the infant's condition is
1. improving.
2. deteriorating.
3. unchanged.
4. uncertain.

58. A 13-year-old boy has an intestinal resection. He has a nasogastric tube that is attached to low, intermittent suction. Two days after surgery, the boy asks the nurse, "When will this tube be taken out?" Which of these responses by the nurse would be accurate?
1. "When you can tolerate fluids by mouth."
2. "When you begin to feel hungry."
3. "When you no longer have gastric drainage."
4. "When you start passing gas rectally."

59. The nurse is helping to develop a teaching plan for a client who is scheduled for a total laryngectomy. It would be *essential* for the plan to include information about which of these topics with respect to the client's early postoperative period?
1. Effects of surgery on facial appearance.
2. Measures to prevent possible wound complications.
3. Anticipated emotional adjustments.
4. Alternate methods of speech.

60. The nurse is teaching a client about ways to promote tissue wound healing after abdominal surgery. The teaching has been effective if the client indicates that she will select foods and beverages that are *high* in which of these vitamins?
1. C
2. D
3. E
4. K_2

61. A client with breast cancer is getting external radiation therapy to the tumor site. Which self-care instruction would be the most important for the nurse to provide?
1. Wear a tight bra to promote maximum support of the breasts.
2. Carefully clean around the port site with warm water each day.
3. Expose the radiation area to sunlight to facilitate healing.
4. Use perfumed deodorant powder to promote a sense of well being.

62. A client has undergone a gastroduodenostomy for treatment of a duodenal ulcer. In teaching him to avoid dumping syndrome, the nurse should instruct him to
1. take warm fluids with meals.
2. eat a high-roughage diet when on full diet.
3. lie down for 30 minutes after each meal.
4. maintain a low-fat, low-carbohydrate diet.

63. A client has been taught about a gastric analysis or gastric acid stimulation test. The client requires *further* teaching if he makes which of these comments?
1. "A small tube will be inserted into my nose."
2. "I will feel heart palpitations for about 10 minutes after I get a medication."
3. "Specimens from my stomach will be collected about every 15 minutes for an hour."
4. "I won't be able to smoke on the morning of the test."

64. A client has a fracture of the right femur and is placed in skeletal traction. Which of these findings, if present, would indicate that the traction was *not* functioning properly?
1. The traction weights rest on the floor.
2. The ropes of the traction are in the grooves of the pulley.
3. There are no pillows supporting the client's affected extremity.
4. The client is in a dorsal recumbent position.

65. A client on the inpatient mental health unit is very suspicious. He does not interact with the other clients and appears to be constantly on his guard. In caring for this client, which of these actions by the nurse is appropriate?
    1. Use gentle, reassuring touch in interactions with him.
    2. Avoid talking with others where the client can see but not hear the conversation.
    3. Ask probing questions during one-to-one interactions with the client.
    4. Prevent the client from spending time alone in his room rather than with other people.

66. A client had a total hip replacement. Two days postoperative, she becomes restless and somewhat confused, and she develops a fine petechial rash over her chest. The nurse should suspect which of these conditions?
    1. Pneumonia
    2. Fat embolism
    3. Pulmonary embolism
    4. Antibiotic sensitivity

67. A male client who has a diagnosis of peptic ulcer attends the clinic. The nurse in the clinic has been having counseling sessions with him. Which of the following statements indicates that he understands what is important in his care?
    1. "I am going to an aerobics class three times a week."
    2. "Instead of snacking on nuts, I'm eating popcorn."
    3. "To relax, I drink a glass or two of wine before going to bed."
    4. "If my stools become tarry in color, I will stop eating foods high in iron."

68. A newborn is admitted to the high-risk nursery after a precipitate birth in the car on the way to the hospital. The infant was exposed to very cold weather and is placed in a radiant warmer. Given this information, the nurse should observe the infant for which of these symptoms?
    1. Episodes of shivering
    2. Cyanosis of the hands and feet
    3. Softness of the fontanels
    4. Periods of apnea

69. A client is to get 0.25 mg of a drug intravenously. The drug is supplied in a vial that has 0.5 mg of the drug in 2 ml of solution. The client should get how many milliliters of the solution?
    1. 0.25
    2. 0.50
    3. 1.0
    4. 1.5

70. A client is getting total parenteral nutrition. While he is getting this treatment, which of these measures should *definitely* be included in his care?
    1. Checking his blood glucose level every 4 to 6 hours.
    2. Maintaining him on bed rest.
    3. Determining the pH of his urine after each voiding.
    4. Keeping him NPO.

THIS IS THE END OF THE PRETEST.

CONTINUE TO THE NEXT PAGE FOR THE CORRECT ANSWERS AND RATIONALE.

ANSWERS AND RATIONALE

Now determine your correct and incorrect choices. For items that you answered correctly, review the rationales to make sure that you got the right answer for the right *reason*. For items that you answered incorrectly, read the rationales and try to determine the reason. Was it because you didn't know the content or was it because you marked an answer incorrectly by mistake?

After you look at each of the rationales, calculate your score and the subscores as explained at the end of the "Answers and Rationales." Evaluate your overall performance on the test. If you got scores below 75% in a category, review content related to that category.

1. Correct answer - 2. Sickle-cell anemia affects many of the body systems and thus is associated with a great variety of symptoms, including painful joints. Options 1, 3, and 4 are not associated with the disease.
CN: Physiological integrity
CA: Pediatric nursing

2. Correct answer - 4. Symptoms of anorexia nervosa include amenorrhea (option 4); bradycardia, rather than tachycardia (option 1); hypotension, rather than increased blood pressure (option 2); and increased physical activity (often, excessive exercise), rather than decreased physical activity (option 4).
CN: Psychosocial integrity
CA: Mental health nursing

3. Correct answer - 2. One of the complications of this procedure is hemorrhage of the puncture site. Thus, the client should be checked frequently for its occurrence. Options 1, 3, and 4: Oral fluids are encouraged to increase urinary output and flush out the dye given during the test; when the catheterization has been performed percutaneously through the femoral artery, the client should remain supine with the affected leg straight and immobile and the head of the bed elevated no more than 30 degrees for several hours.
CN: Safe, effective care environment
CA: Medical/surgical nursing

4. Correct answer - 3. Good sources of potassium include fruits, vegetables, legumes, nuts, whole grains, and meat. A medium banana has about 450 mg of potassium. Options 1, 2, and 4: These contain much less potassium than a banana. For example, a slice of toasted, white bread has 27 mg potassium, a large, boiled egg has 65 mg of potassium and a cup of corn flakes has 30 mg of potassium.
CN: Physiological integrity
CA: Medical/surgical nursing

5. Correct answer - 3. Quickening usually occurs toward the end of the 5th month (18 to 20 weeks) but, at times, can be experienced as early as the 16th or as late as the 22nd week of gestation. Options 1, 2, and 4: These weeks of gestation are outside these limits.
CN: Health promotion and maintenance
CA: Maternity nursing

6. Correct answer - 1. There is breast fullness early in pregnancy. Option 2: If tingling is present as a symptom of pregnancy, it is usually in the breasts. Option 3: Hair loss is not a common symptom prenatally. It may occur in the postpartal period. Option 4: Fatigue, or sleepiness, is a common symptom early in pregnancy.
CN: Health promotion and maintenance
CA: Maternity nursing

7. Correct answer - 1. These are all signs and symptoms of hypokalemia. Options 2, 3, and 4 are all incorrect.
CN: Physiological integrity
CA: Medical/surgical nursing

8. Correct answer - 2. Haldol is neuroleptic of choice for psychotic older adults because it causes fewer anticholinergic side effects, especially

agitation and hyperactivity. Option 1: In doses as low as 20 mg daily, Mellaril can produce an anticholinergic delirium in older adults, especially if the individual has organic brain disorder. Option 3: This is used to treat depression, not psychosis. Option 4: This is used to induce sleep in older adults.
CN: Safe, effective care environment
CA: Mental health nursing

9. Correct answer - 3. One formula to determine the infusion rate is:

$$\frac{\text{Solution volume x drop factor}}{\text{Total time in minutes}} = \text{drops/minute}$$

For example:

$$\frac{3000 \times 15}{1440} = \frac{45000}{1440} = 31.25 \text{ drops/minute}$$

Options 1, 2, and 4 are incorrect.
CN: Physiological integrity
CA: Medical/surgical nursing

10. Correct answer - 1. When a client has heard distressing news, crying is an appropriate reaction and the nurse should remain with her to provide comfort as needed. Option 2: Clients should be allowed to display appropriate behavior. The use of a sedative at this point is premature. Option 3: When a client is obviously distressed is the wrong time to try to get information. Option 4: The client is expressing her feelings by crying and should be allowed to do so.
CN: Psychosocial integrity
CA: Mental health nursing

11. Correct answer - 2. Temporary paralysis of the intestine during the postoperative period may cause distention. To determine if the bowel is functioning, the nurse should listen for bowel sounds. Option 1 and 3: The client should not be given ice and should be encouraged to ambulate. Option 4: Applying a binder will have no effect on eliminating accumulated flatus.
CN: Physiological integrity
CA: Medical/surgical nursing

12. Correct answer - 4. The presence of esophageal atresia is suspected in an infant with excessive salivation and in a newborn with drooling that is frequently accompanied by choking, coughing and cyanosis. Options 1, 2, and 3 are not symptoms of this condition.
CN: Physiological integrity
CA: Pediatric nursing

13. Correct answer - 2. The effectiveness of antipsychotic medication is indicated by a lessening of psychotic symptoms, such as decreased delusions or hallucinations. Option 1: This indicates that symptoms are still present. Option 3: This indicates compliance with the medication regimen, rather than the effectiveness of the medication. Option 4: This describes a common adverse effect (orthostatic hypotension) of antipsychotic medications.
CN: Psychosocial integrity
CA: Mental health nursing

14. Correct answer - 3. Detecting lung cancer in the early stage is difficult. Symptoms such as coughing, blood-streaked sputum, and chest pain occur later. Options 1, 2, and 4: At this time, there is no definite chemotherapeutic treatment for curing the disease; age does not seem to be a factor in the survival rate; and pain is a late sign.
CN: Physiological integrity
CA: Medical/surgical nursing

15. Correct answer - 2. Most pregnant women are given supplementary iron because an ordinary diet does not provide the amount of iron needed during pregnancy. The client's lactovegetarian diet poses an even greater risk for iron deficiency, because it does not include meat or egg yolk, which are excellent sources of iron. Option 1: The client's diet is less likely to be deficient in calcium because it includes milk and cheese. Options 3 and 4: Carotene and ascorbic acid are found in fruits and vegetables, which are included in the client's diet.
CN: Health promotion and maintenance
CA: Maternity nursing

16. Correct answer - 3. Slow reaction to light by the pupils indicates increased intracranial pressure, which also occurs when there is a cerebrovascular accident. Options 1, 2, and 4 generally are not considered initially because the nurse must first know if the intracranial pressure is increased.
CN: Physiological integrity
CA: Medical/surgical nursing

17. Correct answer - 2. Cytoxan has a pronounced immunosuppressive effect and is therefore highly toxic. In addition to the leukocyte count, the platelet count and hematocrit are also important to monitor. Options 1, 3, and 4 are therefore incorrect.
CN: Physiological integrity
CA: Pediatric nursing

18. Correct answer - 2. Although many factors can cause injury to the pancreas, the primary etiological ones are alcoholism and biliary tract disease (i.e., cholecystitis). Because the question is asking *most* likely related, alcoholism is the correct answer. Other less common causes include trauma, viral infections, duodenal ulcer, cysts, abscesses, certain drugs (not antacids though) and certain metabolic disorders (i.e., hyperparathyroidism). Options 1, 3, and 4 are therefore incorrect.
CN: Physiological integrity
CA: Medical/surgical nursing

19. Correct answer - 1. Signs and symptoms of acute left ventricular dysfunction are associated primarily with pulmonary congestion, which is characterized by bilateral, bibasilar crackles. Options 2, 3, and 4 are all signs of right-sided heart failure.
CN: Physiological integrity
CA: Medical/surgical nursing

20. Correct answer - 2. After a transurethral prostatectomy, clients are instructed that because the prostate tissue is removed through the urethra, there may be burning on urination and/or dribbling of urine for a few weeks. Option 1: The client should eat a high-fiber diet to prevent constipation, and hence straining to defecate which could cause hemorrhage. Option 3: Sitting increases intra-abdominal pressure, which could possibly cause

discomfort. Therefore, walking or lying are preferable. Option 4: There is no incision because a resectoscope is inserted into the urethra during the surgery.
CN: Physiological integrity
CA: Medical/surgical nursing

21. Correct answer - 1. Bleeding is a danger sign in pregnancy and may indicate a threatened abortion, especially when accompanied by cramping. The client should be examined promptly to determine the cause of bleeding. Option 3: After examination, if the bleeding is slight, the client may be prescribed bed rest, abstinence from coitus, and perhaps sedation. If bleeding stops, she may undertake limited activities. Options 2 and 4: The client need not lie on the left side, nor is there a need to increase fluid intake.
CN: Health promotion and maintenance
CA: Maternity nursing

22. Correct answer - 2. Two of the earliest symptoms of heart failure are dyspnea and fatigue. Decreased cardiac output results in poor perfusion, manifested by cold extremities, weak pulses, low blood pressure, mottled skin, extreme pallor or duskiness. Options 1 and 4t relevant. Option 3: With systemic venous congestion, weight gain occurs.
CN: Physiological integrity
CA: Pediatric nursing

23. Correct answer - 3. When speaking to a hearing impaired client, face him at his eye level. Option 1: Because difficulty perceiving high tones occurs first among the elderly, using a low-pitched tone of voice is better. Option 2: Speaking directly into a client's ear distorts the message and hides visual cues. Option 4: The best distance for speaking to a hearing-impaired person is 3 to 6 feet.
CN: Safe, effective care environment
CA: Mental health nursing

24. Correct answer - 1
Early adverse effects of Lanoxin include nausea, vomiting and anorexia. Other adverse effects

include drowsiness, apathy, depression, and seeing yellow-green halos around lights. Options 2, 3, and 4 are therefore incorrect.
CN: Safe, effective care environment
CA: Pediatric nursing

25. Correct answer - 2
Bronchiolitis is a relatively common infectious disease of the lower respiratory tract that usually affects children between 2 and 12 months old. The disease usually begins as a simple upper respiratory infection with serous nasal discharge. In addition to fever and cough, other symptoms include dyspnea, irritability, wheezing, tachypnea and intercostal and subcostal retractions. Options 1, 3, and 4 are therefore incorrect.
CN: Safe, effective care environment
CA: Pediatric nursing

26. Correct answer - 3
The nurse may be listening to the uterine souffle, which matches the mother's pulse rate, usually between 60 and 90 bpm. Normal fetal heart rate is 120 to 140 bpm. Option 1: Unless the nurse is sure this is the fetal heart rate, it should not be recorded. Option 2: If there is a low fetal heart rate, a left side-lying position is recommended. Option 4: Because this may not be the fetal heart rate, deep breaths are not necessary. If there is low fetal heart rate, oxygen is given.
CN: Safe, effective care environment
CA: Maternity nursing

27. Correct answer - 4. The initial voided urine is not included in the specimen because it may contain contaminants from the urethra or perineal area. Options 1, 2, and 3: Clients do not need to be NPO; the specimen container should be sterile because the purpose of the testing is to confirm the presence of urinary tract infection and, if present, to identify the causative organism; the perineum should be cleansed with motions that go from the front to the back so that the urinary meatus does not become contaminated with organisms from the anal area.
CN: Safe, effective care environment
CA: Medical/surgical nursing

28. Correct answer - 2. Smoking is associated with premature birth and intrauterine growth retardation of the fetus; small or preterm infants are at greater risk for developmental problems. Option 1: An infant's chance for good health is greater with a reasonably high birth weight. Therefore, a pregnant client should increase (not decrease) caloric intake by approximately 300 calories daily. Option 3: Because smoking is related to having small or preterm infants, option 3 is untrue. Option 4: Any smoking during pregnancy is harmful and should be strongly discouraged.
CN: Health promotion and maintenance
CA: Maternity nursing

29. Correct answer - 1. Myelomeningocele is a defect in which part of the meninges and spinal cord protrude through the vertebral column. Thus, the infant is at risk for developing infections from the area of the defect, which could cause meningitis or encephalitis, and the urinary bladder because these infants commonly require urinary catheterizations and because they frequently lack muscle control of the bladder. Options 2, 3, and 4 are not associated with this particular defect.
CN: Safe, effective care environment
CA: Pediatric nursing

30. Correct answer - 4. Symptoms of adrenal insufficiency (Addison's disease) include low blood pressure. Options 1, 2, and 3 are incorrect as they are all symptoms of excessive adrenocortical hormone secretion (Cushing's syndrome).
CN: Physiological integrity
CA: Medical/surgical nursing

31. Correct answer - 3. Massaging or rubbing the affected limb when a thrombophlebitis is present may dislodge a clot and cause an embolism. Option 1: The affected leg should be elevated to enhance venous return. Option 2: The client will be placed on bed rest to avoid an embolism. Option 4: Warm, moist packs are ordered to gently stimulate circulation.
CN: Physiological integrity
CA: Medical/surgical nursing

32. Correct answer - 2. Soiled linens should be checked to make sure that they do not contain the source of radiation. Options 1, 3, and 4: The container should be lined with lead not aluminum; people who are under 18 years old or who are pregnant or lactating should not visit or care for a client who has internal radiation; these clients are placed on bedrest until the radiation treatment is finished.
CN: Safe, effective care environment
CA: Medical/surgical nursing

33. Correct answer - 1. Seizures are common complications of alcohol withdrawal if detoxification is not managed adequately. Option 2: The client's environment should be quiet, with subdued lighting. Option 3: Fluids should be encouraged, since dehydration and electrolyte imbalance may occur due to diaphoresis and hyperactivity. Option 4: Restraints are usually not used, since they may cause the client to become more agitated.
CN: Psychosocial integrity
CA: Mental health nursing

34. Correct answer - 3. School-age children need contact with children their own age and enjoy playing board games. Option 1: Blocks are more appropriate for preschool children. Option 2: Watching television is a passive diversional activity that does not promote social development. Option 4: The school-age child is capable of reading a book herself.
CN: Health promotion and maintenance
CA: Pediatric nursing

35. Correct answer - 4. Osmitrol, an osmotic diuretic, is prescribed to reduce increased intracranial pressure, which will then reduce cerebral edema. Options 1, 2, and 3: Many diuretics put the client at risk for electrolyte imbalance. While it is true that Osmitrol may be used to prevent or treat the oliguric phase of acute renal failure in some instances, there is no indication that the client has that problem. A diuretic will tend to reduce blood volume rather than increasing it.
CN: Physiological integrity
CA: Medical/surgical nursing

36. Correct answer - 1. The client is likely to be on oxygen therapy, which tends to dry mucous membranes. Additionally, good oral hygiene reduces the risk of infection. Option 2: The use of hydrogen peroxide in the bath is not indicated. Options 3 and 4: The client is likely to have diarrhea and should be encouraged to have high-protein, high-calorie feedings frequently.
CN: Physiological integrity
CA: Medical/surgical nursing

37. Correct answer - 4. Because of the potential diagnosis of impaired skin integrity related to edema, which is common in nephrotic syndrome, an important intervention is to provide meticulous skin care. Option 1: Because of fluid volume excess related to fluid accumulation in tissues, urine needs to be tested for specific gravity and albumin. Option 2: Also because of fluid volume excess, the goal should be to prevent increased fluid intake. Option 3: Because there is the potential for infection related to lowered body defenses, the child should be kept warm and dry.
CN: Physiological integrity
CA: Pediatric nursing

38. Correct answer - 3. The exact deficits from a spinal cord injury are difficult to determine immediately after the injury because of the presence of spinal shock, which results in the complete loss of motor and sensory activity below the level of the lesion. In addition, this client has had an incomplete transection of the cord, which further impedes the ability to accurately predict the exact deficits. With an injury at the level of the first and second lumbar vertebrae, the client may have varying control of his legs and pelvis and some instability in his lower back. Options 1, 2, and 4: It is too early to determine the extent of permanent damage. Unfortunately, the body cannot make new nerve cells.
CN: Physiological integrity
CA: Medical/surgical nursing

39. Correct answer - 4. In the acute phase, it is very important to determine if the client passes the calculus. Therefore, all urine should be strained in an effort to detect the passage of the stone. Options 1, 2, and 3: If compresses are used in an attempt to help relieve pain, they should be *warm,* not cold; the client can assume any position of comfort and should ambulate as much as possible when without pain to encourage passage of the calculus; and finally, fluids are forced (up to 3,000 to 4,000 ml daily) to help in the passage of the calculus.
CN: Safe, effective care environment
CA: Medical/surgical nursing

40. Correct answer - 1. The nurse should check the morphine sulfate order with the health care provider because the route of administration is I.M. rather than I.V. Pain-relieving drugs are given I.V. to provide immediate relief. Also, for the first few days following an MI, intramuscular injections are avoided because they may falsely elevate serum cardiac enzyme levels. Options 2, 3, and 4 are orders typically written for clients with MIs.
CN: Safe, effective care environment
CA: Medical/surgical nursing

41. Correct answer - 4. Right-side-lying position after feeding permits the feeding to flow toward the lower end of the stomach and any swallowed air to rise. Options 1, 2, and 3 are therefore incorrect.
CN: Safe, effective care environment
CA: Pediatric nursing

42. Correct answer - 1. Vasoocclusive (thrombocytic) crisis is the most common type of sickle-cell crisis and is sometimes called painful crisis because of the painful symptoms. Thus, priority should be given to pain relief. Options 2, 3, and 4 can be dealt with at a later time.
CN: Physiological integrity
CA: Pediatric nursing

43. Correct answer - 1. One of the most effective means of liquefying thick sputum is by ensuring that the client has a minimum of 2,000 ml of fluid

daily. Adequate fluid intake thins the client's mucus, which makes it easier to cough up. Therefore, a first step in helping to solve this problem is to determine the client's actual fluid intake. Options 2, 3, and 4: Collecting data about the volume of gas either inspired or exhaled during breathing, which is called tidal volume, whether the client is performing pursed lip breathing exercises, which help improve oxygen transport, or whether the client is placed in Trendelenburg position, will do little to help liquify the client's respiratory secretions and therefore are incorrect.
CN: Safe, effective care environment
CA: Medical/surgical nursing

44. Correct answer - 2. Southeast Asians believe that looking someone in the eye when speaking to them is improper. Option 1: Asians tend to have a sharp separation between the sexes; it is likely to be difficult for an Asian woman to have a male health care provider or nurse. Option 3: Many Asians enter the health care system only reluctantly after all family coping efforts have failed. Option 4: Asians are more likely to enter the health care system with somatic complaints, which are more culturally acceptable than mental health symptoms.
CN: Safe, effective care environment
CA: Mental health nursing

45. Correct answer - 2. The client's assessment data are characteristic of the active phase of labor. Option 1: The latent phase of labor is characterized by cervical dilatation of 0 to 4 cm and contractions every 5 to 20 minutes for 30 to 50 seconds. Option 3: The transitional stage of labor is characterized by cervical dilatation of 8 to 10 cm and contractions every 2 to 3 minutes for 60 to 90 seconds. Option 4: The end of the first stage occurs when the cervix is completely dilated (10 cm) and expulsion of the infant begins.
CN: Health promotion and maintenance
CA: Maternity nursing

46. Correct answer - 4. If a client's kidneys cannot function, he tends to retain fluids, which will be reflected in weight gain. Option 1: The client tends to retain fluids, not to be dehydrated.

Option 2: With chronic renal failure, the life span of RBCs is decreased, erythropoietin is decreased, and folic acid and some blood is lost during dialysis. Decreased--not increased--hemoglobin would be expected. Option 3: A low-protein diet is recommended for patients with renal disease.
CN: Physiological integrity
CA: Medical/surgical nursing

47. Correct answer - 3. To prevent the spread of infection by droplets, the child should be placed on respiratory isolation for at least 24 hours after antibiotic therapy is started. The other types of isolation are not required. Option 1: Enteric, Protective, or Wound and Skin precautions will not prevent infections spread by droplets.
CN: Safe, effective care environment
CA: Pediatric nursing

48. Correct answer - 1. Going out to be with others in church or social gatherings is a sign that resolution is occurring. Options 2 and 3 indicate that the client has not quite accepted the finality of her loss. Option 4 indicates that the client has guilt feelings and blames herself for not preventing her husband's death.
CN: Psychosocial integrity
CA: Mental health nursing

49. Correct answer - 2. Heart failure generally results from a strain on the heart. The ventricles cannot pump enough blood to meet the body's demands. A condition that leads to ventricular overload is hypertension. Option 1: Tight-fitting undergarments do not place extra strain on the heart. Options 3 and 4 are not factors that place people at risk for heart failure.
CN: Physiological integrity
CA: Medical/surgical nursing

50. Correct answer - 3. Some of the symptoms of developmental dysplasia of the hip in an infant include asymmetry of the gluteal and thigh folds, limited hip abduction, apparent femur shortening and Ortolani's sign (audible click during hip abduction and rotation). Although treatment varies with the age of the child and the extent of the

problem, the aim of corrective devices like the Frejka pillow splint, is to hold the dislocated hip in full abduction until a stable joint is produced. When the procedure is successful, the child is able to fully abduct his affected extremity. Options 1, 2, and 4 are incorrect.
CN: Physiological integrity
CA: Pediatric nursing

51. Correct answer - 2. When second-degree burns are present, there has been destruction to the outer layer of skin. Option 1: Blistering, redness and pain are present. Blisters are not present in first-degree burns. Options 3 and 4: There is no pain or blistering in third- and fourth-degree burns.
CN: Physiological integrity
CA: Medical/surgical nursing

52. Correct answer - 4. Encourage the client to express his thoughts and feelings about his situation. Option 1: Dismisses the client's concern and gives false reassurance. Option 2: Diminishes the client's individual concern by casting him as one of thousands. Option 3: Ignores the client's concern and suggests how he should be feeling.
CN: Psychosocial integrity
CA: Mental health nursing

53. Correct answer - 1. Consent is not informed if the client is confused, unconscious, mentally incompetent, or under the influence of sedatives. The client should have been asked to sign the consent form before the medications were given. Because he was not, notify the charge nurse to determine what steps to take next. Option 2, 3, and 4 are therefore incorrect.
CN: Safe, effective care environment
CA: Medical/surgical nursing

54. Correct answer - 1. An adverse effect of Methergine is hypertension. Options 2 and 4: The drug is not associated with the occurrence of hypoglycemia, or urinary retention. Option 3: Methergine stimulates strong uterine contractions, not uterine atony.
CN: Health promotion and maintenance
CA: Maternity nursing

55. Correct answer - 3. Before an analgesic is administered, the urinary drainage system should be checked for patency because an obstructed system can cause pain. Options 1, 2, and 4: Following a TUR, the Credé maneuver, which helps to empty the urinary bladder, is contraindicated. Determining when the client last had pain medication or repositioning him can be done after the patency of his catheter is checked.
CN: Physiological integrity
CA: Medical/surgical nursing

56. Correct answer - 1. Common adverse effects of Dilantin include drowsiness, hirsutism, nystagmus, and hyperplasia of the gum. The urine may turn pink, red or brown. Options 2, 3, and 4 are incorrect.
CN: Physiological integrity
CA: Medical/surgical nursing

57. Correct answer - 1. The Apgar score is calculated by adding the scores of each of the 5 observed signs on a scale from 0 to 2. A heart rate over 100 is scored 2; a respiratory effort of "good and crying" is scored 2; muscle tone of "some flexion of extremities" is scored 1; reflex irritability of "weak cry" is scored 1; and color of "body pink, extremities blue" is scored 1, for a total score of 7. The increased Apgar score indicates that the infant is improving. Options 2, 3, and 4 are therefore incorrect.
CN: Health promotion and maintenance
CA: Maternity nursing

58. Correct answer - 4. Gastric decompression continues until there is evidence of intestinal activity, such as the passing of flatus rectally or of stool. Options 1, 2, and 3 do not indicate specifically that intestinal activity is occurring.
CN: Physiological integrity
CA: Pediatric nursing

59. Correct answer - 4. In this type of surgery, the vocal cords are removed, which means that the client will not be able to speak. The inability to make one's needs known can be *very* frightening. Therefore, the nurse must discuss alternate methods of communication with the client. Options 1, 2, and 3: While these topics are important, they are not *essential*. To a large extent, teaching the client about these topics depends on his concerns and readiness to learn about them preoperatively.
CN: Safe, effective care environment
CA: Medical/surgical nursing

60. Correct answer - 1. Vitamin C's significant role in cementing the ground substance of supportive tissue makes it an important agent in wound healing. This creates extra demands for vitamin C in traumatic injury or surgery, especially where extensive tissue regeneration is required. Options 2, 3, and 4: Vitamin D plays an important role in regulating bone mineral (i.e., calcium and phosphorus) metabolism; vitamin E, in hemopoiesis; and vitamin K_2, in blood clotting.
CN: Physiological integrity
CA: Medical/surgical nursing

61. Correct answer - 2. The markings of the radiation (port) site need to be retained and should not be washed off. Neither hot nor cold temperatures should come in contact with the skin exposed to radiation. Option 1: Restrictive clothing should be avoided. Option 3: The potentially dry skin of the radiation site should not be exposed to the sun. Option 4: Perfume and powders should be avoided because of their drying and irritating potential.
CN: Health promotion and planning
CA: Medical/surgical nursing

62. Correct answer - 3. Lying down lessens dumping syndrome by permitting better blood distribution to the gastrointestinal tract during the early digestive processes. Option 1: Treatment of dumping syndrome includes not taking fluids with meals. Options 2 and 4: A high-protein, high-fat, low-carbohydrate, dry diet is given to alleviate dumping syndrome.
CN: Health promotion and maintenance
CA: Medical/surgical nursing

63. Correct answer - 2. During this test, clients are given histamine or betazole (Histalog) to

stimulate gastric secretions. After the medication is injected, the client probably will have a *flushed* feeling. Because palpitations are not typical, the client's knowledge of this aspect needs to be discussed further. Options 1, 3, and 4: All of these measures should occur during a gastric analysis. Thus, the client has understood these parts of the instructions.
CN: Safe, effective care environment
CA: Medical/surgical nursing

64. Correct answer - 1. The weights of the traction should be hanging freely, not resting on the bed or the floor as this negates the effect of the traction. When the weights are on the floor, the traction is not functioning properly and corrective action is required. Options 2, 3, and 4: The ropes should move freely through the grooves in the pulley. Usually, no pillow is placed under the affected extremity because a pillow may counteract the effects of traction. The client usually lies flat.
CN: Safe, effective care environment
CA: Medical/surgical nursing

65. Correct answer - 2. When a suspicious client sees other people talking, he mistakenly assumes that the people are talking about him ("ideas of reference"). The nurse should avoid such situations because they reinforce the client's suspicion. Option 1: Touch is perceived as a threat by suspicious clientss and should be avoided. A suspicious client should be allowed to control the amount of self-revelation that takes place in the interactions with the nurse. Option 3: A probing approach will only alienate the client. Since suspicious people fear intrusion from others and question their motives, care must be taken to respect the client's right to privacy. Option 4: Time alone should be worked into the client's daily schedule.
CN: Psychosocial integrity
CA: Mental health nursing

66. Correct answer - 2. Fat embolism can occur from surgical trauma and petechial rash is a major sign of this complication. Options 1 and 3: Rash is not a usual symptom of pneumonia or pulmonary

embolism. Option 4: Antibiotic rashes generally occur over the entire body.
CN: Safe, effective care environment
CA: Medical/surgical nursing

67. Correct answer - 1. Exercise is a good stress management technique and helps alleviate frustration. The cause of gastric ulcers seems to be related to stress. Popcorn, nuts, and alcohol are generally eliminated from the diet. Therefore, options 2 and 3 are incorrect. Option 4: Tarry stools are a sign of bleeding and should be reported immediately.
CN: Physiological integrity
CA: Medical/surgical nursing

68. Correct answer - 4. The infant has experienced cold stress and is being rewarmed. Rapid warming may cause apneic spells and acidosis in an infant. Option 1: Newborns do not shiver. Option 2: Cyanosis of the hands and feet (acrocyanosis) is normally found in the newborn. Option 3: Assessment of the fontanels is not relevant to cold stress.
CN: Health promotion and maintenance
CA: Maternity nursing

69. Correct answer - 3. One way to calculate dosage is the proportion method. Using this method:

$$\frac{0.25 \text{ mg}}{x} = \frac{0.5 \text{ mg}}{2 \text{ ml}}$$
$$0.5\,x = 0.50$$
$$x = 1 \text{ ml}$$

Options 1, 2, and 4 are incorrect.
CN: Physiological integrity
CA: Medical/surgical nursing

70. Correct answer - 1. Solutions used in total parenteral nutrition contain a lot of glucose to increase caloric intake. The pancreas must adapt to the increased glucose in the circulation by producing more insulin. To determine how well the pancreas is adapting to the increased load of glucose, blood (or urine, if blood testing means are not available) is tested on a routine basis (every 4 to 6 hours). In this way, complications resulting

from either hyperglycemia or hypoglycemia can be averted. Options 2, 3, and 4: None of these measures *definitely* needs to be included in a client's care. Determining the pH of the urine is not relevant in this situation and, depending on the individual situation, many clients are allowed or encouraged to ambulate, in fact, encouraged, and to eat or drink.
CN: Safe, effective care environment
CA: Medical/surgical nursing

PERSONAL DIAGNOSTIC PROFILE   (see the following page for instructions)

QUESTION NUMBER																				Totals

TEST-TAKING SKILLS

Misread the question																				
Missed important point																				
Forgot fact or concept																				
Applied wrong fact or concept																				
Drew wrong conclusion																				
Incorrectly evaluated distractors																				
Mistakenly selected answer choice																				
Read into question																				
Made a wrong guess																				
Misunderstood question																				

CLIENT NEED CATEGORIES

Safe, effective care environment																				
Physiological integrity																				
Psychosocial integrity																				
Health promotion and maintenance																				

CLINICAL AREAS

Pediatric nursing																				
Maternity nursing																				
Medical/surgical nursing																				
Mental health nursing																				

HOW TO SCORE AND USE THE DIAGNOSTIC PROFILE

In the top "QUESTION NUMBER" row of boxes, mark each question number you answered wrong. Under each question number, check the box in the "TEST TAKING SKILLS" section that is the most appropriate reason you answered the question incorrectly. Do the same for the "CLIENT NEED CATEGORIES" AND "CLINICAL AREAS" section. The client need and clinical area codes follow the rationale. Total the number of check marks, by line, in the "Totals" column. This provides you with a profile of your weak areas that should be improve upon prior to taking the NCLEX-RN.

CALCULATION OF SUBSCORES

After you score your test, determine your subscores in these areas by filling in the following two grids.

CLINICAL AREA

	Medical/Surgical nursing	Pediatric nursing	Maternity nursing	Mental health nursing
Number of questions	36	14	10	10
Number incorrect				
Number correct				
Percent correct*				

*To determine the percent correct, divide the number of items answered correctly by the total number of items and multiply the results by 100.

CLIENT NEED

	Safe, effective care environment	Physiological integrity	Psychosocial integrity	Health promotion & maintenance
Number of questions	21	30	7	12
Number incorrect				
Number correct				
Percent correct*				

*To determine the percent correct in each category, divide the number of items answered correctly by the total number of items and multiply the result by 100.

Note: This is a short test with a limited sample of items in each category. Therefore, if a score in any category is less than 75% correct, further study is strongly advised.

CHAPTER 3

Mental Health Nursing Skill Test

TAKING THIS SKILL TEST

Your Study Guide Module has instructed you to take the following skill test after you have completed your review of the clinical area. This test will give you needed experience in answering NCLEX-RN type questions and will give you a good idea of your competence in this clinical area.

The format of the skill test gives you instant feedback as you take it. Each question is in the left column. The correct answer with rationale is in the right column. As you read the question in the left-hand column, cover the right-hand column with an index card until you have selected your answer. Slide the card down, keeping remaining question answers covered. When you have completed the test, use the Personal Diagnostic Profile to record why you answered any question incorrectly.

If you scored lower than 75% on this skill test, you should analyze the reason and go back and do further review. You may also wish to consult a current nursing textbook for any areas that are unclear to you.

1. An actively manic client has been on Lithobid (lithium carbonate) for 5 days. She frequently enters other clients' rooms and takes their possessions, claiming they belong to her. She becomes irate if she has to wait for anything. One day she throws her arms around her nurse, gives her a big wet kiss on the cheek, and says, "You are my most favorite nurse of all times." What would be the priority nursing diagnosis for this client?
   1. Impaired verbal communication related to mania.
   2. Impaired adjustment related to invading others boundaries.
   3. Risk for violence to others related to impulsiveness.
   4. Altered thought processes related to claiming possessions as her own.

2. The nurse is explaining to a family how to manage the care of their loved one who has mania. The family asks how they will know when to seek treatment for their loved one. The nurse instructs them to seek help if he
   1. becomes socially active.
   2. displays anger when frustrated.
   3. expresses displeasure with having to take medication.
   4. becomes impulsive or increases his use of alcohol.

3. The nursing needs of an acutely manic person should be prioritized according to
   1. functional level of the client.
   2. amount of stimulation in the environment.
   3. length of time the client has been manic.
   4. amount of lithium administered.

4. A manic client uses sexually explicit language with opposite sex clients and staff. The best way for the nurse to deal with this client is to
   1. explain he is inappropriate; help him rephrase his comments.
   2. put him on a behavior contract; post it for all to see.
   3. help him process his need to use seductive language.
   4. ask him what he hopes to accomplish by this behavior.

1. Correct answer - 3. Any actively manic person has poor impulse control and therefore, a risk for harming self or others. Option 1: Verbal communication is not impaired and the etiology statement contains a medical diagnosis. Options 2 and 4: The etiology statements for these are incorrect.
CN: Psychosocial integrity

2. Correct answer - 4. This indicates the return of symptoms and is correct. None of the remaining options indicate manic behaviors, but normal responses to various stimuli.
CN: Psychosocial integrity

3. Correct answer - 1. Level of functioning dictates type of nursing intervention as well as indicates any safety needs. Options 2, 3, and 4 have nothing to do with priorities for nursing needs.
CN: Psychosocial integrity

4. Correct answer - 1. This provides the client with feedback and structure. Options 2, 3, and 4 assume that the client is able to thoughtfully consider his actions. Being actively manic, he cannot. Behavior contracts work with people who are able to control their behavior.
CN: Psychosocial integrity

5. A client has a blood alcohol content of 0.27 on admission to the psychiatric unit. Fifteen hours later, it would most likely be
   1. 0.00
   2. 0.12
   3. 0.027
   4. 0.012

6. You recognize that one of your nursing colleagues is impaired by alcohol abuse. You decide to take over some of her work for her. Your behavior illustrates the concept of
   1. being responsible to.
   2. unconditional positive regard.
   3. co-dependency.
   4. enabling.

7. An alcoholic client says he has blackouts regularly and can consume a fifth of alcohol a day without feeling inebriated. He says he usually consumes from mid-afternoon to bedtime and that his drinking allows him to "not get too uptight," as he is in a high stress job. Where would this client fall on the Alcohol Consumption Continuum?
   1. End stage
   2. Late dependency
   3. Middle dependency
   4. Early dependency

8. You and several colleagues decide to intervene with a colleague who is chemically impaired. What is the *first* step you should take?
   1. Contact an intervention counselor for assistance.
   2. Determine what key people are willing to participate.
   3. Set up a meeting with the impaired colleague.
   4. Make a list of what you want to say to your colleague.

5. Correct answer - 2. Alcohol is cleared from the body at the rate of .01 per hour. To compute the answer, subtract .15 from .27. The person will be cleared of alcohol in 27 hours. The other options would be incorrect levels based on alcohol elimination formula.
CN: Physiological integrity

6. Correct answer - 4. An enabler supports another's behaviors so that the person is spared experiencing consequences. Option 1: Being responsible to means being available to the person, *not* rescuing her. Option 2: The nurse values the other person, it does not mean covering up for her. Option 3: Co-dependency is defined as finding one's own identity by trying to control outcomes.
CN: Psychosocial integrity

7. Correct answer - 3. This is the correct choice. Options 1 and 2 are the same. In late dependency, the individual consumes to feel "normal" and there is liver damage. Option 4: In early dependency, the individual may have only an occasional blackout and tolerance is still building. Excessive *daily* drinking is generally not the pattern.
CN: Psychosocial integrity

8. Correct answer - 1. The counselor can help the people involved determine who should participate, what to say, and how to say it. After the "players" are in place and are clear about how to confront their colleague, someone will arrange a time for the direct intervention to occur. Options 2, 3, and 4 would all happen *after* contacting the counselor.
CN: Safe, effective care environment

9. A client who is recovering from alcohol abuse has not had a drink for 2 weeks, complains of many bodily discomforts, and demonstrates a marked decrease in her ability to tolerate stress. Which of the following phenomena is this client demonstrating?
   1. Decreased tolerance
   2. Withdrawal syndrome
   3. Korsakoff's syndrome
   4. Abstinence syndrome

9. Correct answer - 4. Abstinence syndrome is characterized by preoccupation with bodily sensations and decreased ability to tolerate stress. Option 1: Decreased tolerance occurs when the individual experiences adverse symptoms with a small amount of alcohol. Option 2: Withdrawal syndrome is a physiological response to not using. Option 3: Korsakoff's syndrome results from thiamine deficiency.
CN: Psychosocial integrity

10. A client enters the emergency department experiencing a "bad trip" from ingesting LSD. What is the best *initial* action for the nurse to take?
    1. Stay with the client and talk him down.
    2. Let the person be alone so he can calm down.
    3. Apply soft restraints so he will not hurt himself or others.
    4. Help the person describe the conditions under which he ingested the drug.

10. Correct answer - 1. The client will respond to the presence of the nurse and will need constant reorientation. Option 2: The client will become more frightened and out of control if left alone. Option 3 may cause him to panic. Option 4 is not a beneficial *first* action because he is most likely not able to process.
CN: Psychosocial integrity

11. A friend whom you know to be overly compulsive and concerned with ritualistically carrying out minor daily routines asks you what he can do about this. Which of the following would be your *best* advice?
    1. Learn meditation skills.
    2. Seek a behavioral therapist's services.
    3. See his health care provider for medication to relieve his anxiety.
    4. Avoid stressful situations.

11. Correct answer - 2. Individuals with obsessive/compulsive disorder (O/CD) respond well to behavioral therapy. Option 1 would be more useful for individuals with generalized anxiety disorder (GAD). Option 3: Medications are not first action of choice. Option 4: No one can avoid stressful situations.
CN: Psychosocial integrity

12. A client, brought to the emergency department has had recurrent nightmares, feels jittery all the time, will not leave her apartment, and startles easily. A friend who accompanied her says the client had been in a fast food restaurant 2 months ago when a person entered and shot customers, killing 4 and wounding 10 others. The client's symptoms have been escalating over the past few weeks. What is this client experiencing?
    1. Agoraphobia
    2. Panic disorder with agoraphobia
    3. Post-traumatic stress disorder
    4. Social phobia

12. Correct answer - 3. The symptoms described are classic for post-traumatic stress disorder. Options 1, 2, and 4 are wrong.
CN: Psychosocial integrity

13. Compared to clients with schizophrenia, clients with anxiety disorders
    1. have fewer ego strengths from which to draw.
    2. are generally more negative in their self-appraisals.
    3. have poorer coping skills and consequently higher level of anxiety.
    4. score higher on the Global Assessment of Function Scale.

13. Correct answer - 4. People with anxiety disorders are generally much more able to meet life demands than people with schizophrenia. Option 1: People with anxiety disorders are functional because of possessing many ego strengths. Option 2: People with anxiety disorders generally have negative self-appraisals about specific things. Option 3: Coping skills are better developed in individuals with anxiety disorders and cognitive processes are generally intact.
CN: Psychosocial integrity

14. A 45-year-old man was admitted to a cardiac unit 10 hours ago, following an episode of chest pain at work that morning. Since admission, the client has had no further chest pain, ECG is within normal limits, and liver enzymes are normal. The client is tremulous, did not eat much lunch or dinner, is restless and sometimes disoriented. His pulse rate is 112 and he is diaphoretic. At the present time, he is receiving no medications. He has asked for some Valium to help him relax. What is the best action for the nurse to take?
    1. Ask the health care provider for a prn order for Valium.
    2. Check his vital signs every 15 minutes.
    3. Remain with him until his anxiety level decreases.
    4. Recommend that he be transferred to a detoxification unit.

14. Correct answer - 4. The client is demonstrating classic signs of alcohol withdrawal and needs to be transferred to a detoxification unit equipped to help him detoxify. Option 1 is not the best choice because although Valium is used to detoxify, it must be carefully calibrated. Option 2 does not help the client detoxify. His pulse will continue to be elevated. Option 3: Anxiety is not the problem here, withdrawal is.
CN: Physiological integrity

15. Anxiety is considered to be pathological when
    1. it reaches panic level.
    2. selective inattention is apparent.
    3. it prohibits the person from enjoying life.
    4. the person exhibits physiological symptoms.

15. Correct answer - 3. Pathological anxiety interferes with one's ability to enjoy life. Option 1: Panic level anxiety can be an appropriate response to a life-threatening situation. Option 2: Selective inattention is associated with moderate level anxiety as well as in fatigue and boredom. Option 4: Physiological symptoms do not necessarily mean anxiety is inappropriate to the situation.
CN: Psychosocial integrity

16. The difference between individuals with panic level anxiety and severe level anxiety is that people with
    1. panic level anxiety have difficulty with reality.
    2. severe anxiety can describe their experience.
    3. severe anxiety benefit from progressive relaxation.
    4. panic level anxiety have problems with selective inattention.

16. Correct answer - 1. This statement is correct. Option 2 is not true. Option 3 is not possible for someone whose anxiety level is severe. Option 4 applies to people with moderate level anxiety.
CN: Psychosocial integrity

17. A nurse is caring for an 80-year-old client who has difficulty dressing appropriately, is periodically incontinent of urine, and frequently gets confused about where her room is. What overriding concept should the nurse keep in mind as she provides care for this client?
    1. Consistency
    2. Role reversal
    3. Developmental stage behavior
    4. Countertransference

17. Correct answer - 1. This client has Alzheimer's disease and needs routine and consistency to remain functional. Option 2: The nurse is not in a role reversal with the client, although the family might be. Option 3: This client's behavior is inconsistent with developmental stage. Option 4: Counter-transference is not the *overriding* concept.
CN: Psychosocial integrity

18. You are the nurse admitting an 85-year-old adult to the long-term-care unit. You should, *initially*
    1. administer standardized psychological tests.
    2. have the person describe events from childhood.
    3. get most information from the client's relatives.
    4. ask the person to describe events in the last 2 days.

18. Correct answer - 4. This lets the nurse assess recent memory as a means of ruling out dementia and assessing the credibility of the information the client gives. Option 1: Psychologists generally do diagnostic testing. Option 2: Remote memory remains intact. Option 3 is needed when the client is deemed unreliable to provide accurate information.
CN: Psychosocial integrity

19. An effective technique for enhancing the *functional level* of a client with early-stage Alzheimer's disease is to
    1. introduce the person to new, solitary activities.
    2. teach the person how to successfully confabulate.
    3. have the person join an Alzheimer's support group.
    4. post a daily routine schedule for the person to follow.

19. Correct answer - 4. A posted schedule provides the person with the structure needed at this stage of the illness. Option 1: Individuals with Alzheimer's find new activities threatening. Option 2: Confabulation is an unconscious defense mechanism and cannot be taught. Option 3: While a support group might help the person grieve, it will not keep him functional.
CN: Psychosocial integrity

20. An 80-year-old client looks into a mirror while brushing her teeth, and screams. "Who is that person staring at me?" What would be a reasonable inference to make about this woman's behavior? She is
    1. hallucinating.
    2. confused and disoriented.
    3. exhibiting agnosia.
    4. agitated.

20. Correct answer - 3. Agnosia is the inability to recognize correctly sensory impressions. This client does not recognize the familiar--her own image. Options 1, 2, and 4 are not correct.
CN: Psychosocial integrity

21. The *major* nursing concern for any client with dementia is
    1. safety.
    2. cognitive functioning.
    3. social appropriateness.
    4. wandering.

21. Correct answer - 1. Any client whose judgment is impaired and who cannot process external cues is at risk for harming self or others, so safety needs supersede all other needs. Options 2, 3, and 4 are concerns, but safety is the major concern.
CN: Safe, effective care environment

22. A priority assessment to do on any adult older than 60 is a
    1. family/social history.
    2. physical assessment.
    3. mental status examination.
    4. neurological examination.

22. Correct answer 3. Organic process such as dementia should be ruled out for any older adult so that appropriate nursing measures can be planned. Options 1, 2, and 4 need to be done, but a mental status examination is essential.
CN: Psychosocial integrity

23. A client had a modified radical mastectomy 3 days ago. Her dressing has just been changed and her drainage tubes removed. She states to the nurse, "Did you see my huge, red incision and the holes left from the drains? It looks horrible!" Which of these responses by the nurse would be appropriate?
    1. "Your incision is inflamed now, but in several weeks it will decrease and the skin will look better."
    2. "Although it's difficult, you must be strong and learn to accept and cope with the changed appearance of your body."
    3. "Your incision actually looks very good, considering the extensive surgery that was performed."
    4. "Many women have this type of surgery and they are not usually so upset."

23. Correct answer - 1. The long incision of a mastectomy can be very unsightly and upsetting to the client. She needs to know that, in time, redness, swelling, and irregularity of the incision will decrease, the scar will become less prominent, and tissues will become more normal in color. Option 2 is not supportive and tells the client how she should feel. Option 3 does not respond to the client's concern about her appearance. Option 4 belittles this client's concerns and feelings rather than dealing with them.
CN: Psychosocial integrity

24. What would be the best nursing diagnosis to enter on a severely depressed client's care plan?
    1. Social isolation related to anhedonia.
    2. Self-care deficit related to ego disintegration.
    3. Fatigue related to staying in bed with eyes closed.
    4. Impaired social interaction related to lack of energy.

24. Correct answer - 4. Depressed people do not have the energy to extend themselves. Option 1: Social isolation is imposed by others, it is *not* self-imposed. Option 2: Poor grooming is an evidence of self-care deficit, not a cause. Option 3: Staying in bed with eyes closed is an evidence of fatigue, not a cause of fatigue.
CN: Psychosocial integrity

25. What is the best way for a nurse to be protected in the event of a lawsuit?
    1. Adhere to agency policies and procedures.
    2. Adequately document own, other's and client's behaviors.
    3. Follow health care provider's order with great precision.
    4. Check with a supervisor before doing questionable procedures.

25. Correct answer - 2. If it's not documented, it didn't happen. A court of law does not accept memory as valid. Option 1 may not always be true. Option 3: A nurse has legal responsibility for assuring orders are accurate and safe. An order could be wrong. Option 4 looks reasonable, but the nurse is always accountable for any actions she carries out.
CN: Safe, effective care environment

26. A male nurse worked with a female client in the psychiatric hospital about 6 months ago. He ran into her at a restaurant and they had a great social time. The woman asks the nurse if they could work on developing a relationship. What would be the *best* response for the nurse to make?
    1. "We can see how things go."
    2. "Nurses and former clients should not become overly friendly."
    3. "I enjoyed this evening, but I do not wish to meet again."
    4. "What kind of commitment are you asking me for?"

26. Correct answer - 3. This sets a clear limit and the nurse took responsibility for his decision. Options 1 and 4 are vague and inconclusive. Option 2 begs the issue and is judgmental.
CN: Safe, effective care environment

27. A client is admitted to the detoxification unit because of alcohol abuse. On admission, it would be *essential* to obtain the answer to which of these questions?
    1. How long has the client been drinking alcohol?
    2. Has the client ever been in an alcohol treatment program?
    3. When did the client have his last drink of alcohol?
    4. Does the client have blackouts while drinking alcohol?

27. Correct answer - 3. When a client abuses alcohol or other substances, tolerance can develop. If alcohol is not available, the client may suffer alcohol withdrawal syndrome. Knowing when the client had his last drink can help to estimate when the symptoms associated with the syndrome are likely to occur and appropriate interventions taken. Options 1, 2, and 4: Although obtaining the answers to these questions on admission is important, learning when the last drink was taken is *most* important.
CN: Psychosocial integrity

28. An adolescent made a suicide attempt after learning his parents were divorcing and that he was not accepted at the college where he had applied. What should the nurse *initially* focus on with this adolescent?
    1. Help him redefine college and career goals.
    2. Identify present and future positives in his life.
    3. Help him accept his parents impending divorce.
    4. Explore options for dealing with things out of his control.

28. Correct answer - 4. This empowers the adolescent to take action on his own behalf to overcome helplessness. Options 1, 2, and 3 are premature interventions initially.
    CN: Safe, effective care environment

29. An elderly, confused client in a long-term-care facility wanders into other clients' rooms, frightening them. Which of these actions would be appropriate for the nurse to take *initially?*
    1. Ask the client why he is wandering.
    2. Secure the client in a vest restraint.
    3. Provide a safe area for the client to wander.
    4. Administer haloperidol (Haldol) as prescribed for the client.

29. Correct answer - 3. As an initial action, the nurse should provide a safe area for wandering to permit exercise and minimize the risk of injury. Option 1: Questioning the behavior is not likely to provide any usable information. Options 2 and 4: Physical restraints or chemical restraints should not be used unless absolutely necessary.
    CN: Safe, effective care environment

30. The *best* outcome criterion for a person with post-traumatic stress disorder (PTSD) would be
    1. ability to avoid trigger events.
    2. cognitive mastery of the traumatic event.
    3. forgiving the person who caused the trauma.
    4. reduction in the occurrence of symptoms.

30. Correct answer - 2. Until cognitive mastery is achieved, the person cannot heal from PTSD. Option 1: Trigger events may not be avoidable nor always identified. Option 3: The trauma may not have been caused by a person. Option 4 is not the best outcome and "reduction" cannot be objectively measured.
    CN: Psychosocial integrity

31. The client has a nursing diagnosis of *self-care deficit related to ritualistic behavior*. Which nursing intervention would be best for this client?
    1. A flexible daily schedule.
    2. Strict adherence to a daily schedule.
    3. Close monitoring to prevent ritualistic behaviors.
    4. A written contract penalizing ritualistic behaviors.

31. Correct answer - 1. The schedule needs to be flexed around rituals, once these have begun. Options 2, 3, and 4: Rituals serve to relieve intolerable anxiety and should not be interrupted once begun and cannot be "pre-scheduled."
    CN: Psychosocial integrity

32. Which of the following is *most* likely to be
found in clients experiencing acute mania?
    1. Social inappropriateness
    2. Hypersomnia and anorexia
    3. Anhedonia and emotional lability
    4. Increased libido and guilt

33. A severely depressed client has responded to
antidepressant therapy and his energy level has
increased. Which of these measures would be
most important to include in his plan of care?
    1. Institute a program of vigorous physical
    activity.
    2. Provide the client with foods high in
    carbohydrate.
    3. Observe the client for suicidal behavior.
    4. Monitor the client's blood pressure.

34. The nurse notices that a client who has been
receiving haloperidol (Haldol) for the past 3
weeks has developed fatigue, weakness, and a
decreased interest in activities that were
formerly satisfying. A reasonable inference
would be that the client
    1. has not been taking the Haldol.
    2. has developed a tolerance to the Haldol.
    3. is having an allergic reaction to the Haldol.
    4. may be receiving too much Haldol.

35. Which time is best to administer phenelzine
(Nardil)?
    1. One hour before meals.
    2. In a loaded bedtime dose.
    3. B.i.d. or t.i.d. with last dose by 3 p.m.
    4. After the evening meal.

36. A 30-year-old woman with bipolar disorder
plans to run in a marathon. She has been taking
lithium since her discharge from the hospital 3
months ago. Running in the marathon puts her
at risk for
    1. akathisia.
    2. return of symptoms.
    3. cholinergic adverse effects.
    4. toxicity.

32. Correct answer - 1. Individuals who are acutely
manic are impulsive and have grossly impaired
judgment. They are often socially
inappropriate. Options 2, 3, and 4:
Hypersomnia, loss of appetite, anhedonia, and
guilt are not behaviors characteristic of mania.
CN: Psychosocial integrity

33. Correct answer - 3. A client is at particular risk
for suicide when he appears to be coming out of
his depression because he may then have the
energy and opportunity to carry out the act.
Option 1: The client is not likely to have
sufficient energy for vigorous physical activity.
Option 2: There is no indication that the client
requires foods high in carbohydrate; he is not in
a manic phase. Option 4: Although postural
hypotension is an adverse effect of some
antidepressants, the most important concern is
the increased risk of suicide.
CN: Psychosocial integrity

34. Correct answer - 4. These are symptoms typical
of overdose. Option 1: The client would not
have these symptoms if not taking the drug.
Option 2: Tolerance to neuroleptics does not
occur. Option 3: Allergic reactions take the
form of rash or breathing problems.
CN: Safe, effective care environment

35. Correct answer - 3. Monoamine oxidase
inhibitors (MAOIs) interfere with sleep, so the
last dose should be no later than 3 or 4 p.m.
Options 1, 2, and 4 would interfere with sleep.
CN: Safe, effective care environment

36. Correct answer - 4. Loss of body fluids leads to
Lithium toxicity. Option 1: Akathisia is an
adverse effect associated with neuroleptics.
Option 2: Overhydration can lead to diluting
lithium in the body, leading to return of manic
symptoms. Option 3 does not apply.
CN: Safe, effective care environment

37. The nurse is doing a suicide assessment on a client and discovers that he has an unstable lifestyle, abuses alcohol, has made one previous suicide attempt on diazepam (Valium), and has ideas for a potential suicide plan which he is still formulating. The nurse assesses this individual's suicide risk to be
    1. low.
    2. high.
    3. moderate.
    4. borderline.

37. Correct answer - 3. Symptoms described are typical of moderate level suicide risk. Option 1: History of a previous attempt would make him greater, not lower risk. Option 2: The stated fact that he is still formulating a plan reduces a high-risk potential. Option 4: There is no borderline category.
CN: Safe, effective care environment

38. Manifestation of anticholinergic adverse effects of neuroleptics include
    1. dry mouth, blurred vision, urinary retention.
    2. lowered WBC count, high fever, sore throat.
    3. confusion, renal failure, bradycardia.
    4. fluctuating vital signs, edema, diaphoresis.

38. Correct answer - 1. These adverse effects are correct. Options 2, 3, and 4 do not reflect anticholinergic adverse effects.
CN: Physiological integrity

39. Which drug is distributed throughout body fluids as a salt when ingested?
    1. Zoloft (Sertraline)
    2. Lithobid (Lithium carbonate)
    3. Clozaril (Clozapine)
    4. Risperdal (Risperidone)

39. Correct answer - 2. Lithobid is the correct choice. Options 1, 3, and 4 are not distributed as salts in the body fluids.
CN: Physiological integrity

40. Which medication is classified as an MAOI?
    1. Amitriptyline (Elavil)
    2. Bupropion (Wellbutrin)
    3. Tranylcypromine (Parnate)
    4. Trazodone (Desyrel)

40. Correct answer - 3. This is the only correct answer.
CN: Physiological integrity

41. A nurse in a long-term-care facility is using remotivation and behavior modification techniques to stimulate a group of regressed elderly clients. Which of these outcomes suggests that the techniques are effective?
    1. Residents are able to start and play games they have been taught.
    2. Residents are able to perform simple activities without thought.
    3. Residents don't discuss their past.
    4. Residents are able to sit and listen to instructions given to them.

41. Correct answer - 1. The ability to participate in and initiate newly learned activities indicates that the residents are based in the present and dealing with reality. Options 2 and 3 do not relate to re-motivation and behavior modification techniques. Option 4: Although residents may be listening to instructions, there is no indication that they are following the instructions.
CN: Psychosocial integrity

42. The nurse is teaching nursing assistants about lithium carbonate. While discussing lithium toxicity, he teaches that lithium toxicity can be precipitated by
    1. fluid restriction.
    2. ingestion of tyramine containing foods.
    3. sharp increase in sodium intake.
    4. fluid overload.

42. Correct answer - 1. The drug is excreted, virtually unchanged, in the urine. Fluid restriction could cause a build-up of the drug in the body, leading to toxicity. Option 2 is associated with MAOI drugs. Option 3: Increased sodium intake does not precipitate toxicity. Option 4: With fluid overload, lithium level would be diluted, causing return of symptoms.
    CN: Physiological integrity

43. The nurse is educating her client, who is taking an MAOI, about tyramine-containing foods. Which foods should the nurse teach the client to avoid?
    1. Salami and bologna
    2. Whole milk and cream cheese
    3. Homemade gravies
    4. White fish and rice

43. Correct answer - 1. Salami and bologna contain tyramine. Options 2, 3, and 4 do not contain tyramine.
    CN: Safe, effective care environment

44. Which of the following findings, noted during a nursing assessment, would alert the nurse that an increase in the dose of a prescribed neuroleptic drug would be needed to control symptoms of mental illness?
    1. Client with diabetes taking insulin
    2. Cigarette smoker
    3. Coexistence of a physical illness
    4. Daily alcohol user

44. Correct answer - 2. Smoking increases the amount of neuroleptic drug needed to achieve the same therapeutic benefit. Options 1, 3, and 4: None of these increases the amount of neuroleptic needed.
    CN: Physiological integrity

45. A client taking a neuroleptic suddenly rolls his eyes upward and remain in a fixed position. The nurse assesses that the client is experiencing
    1. torticollis.
    2. nystagmus.
    3. opisthotonos.
    4. oculogyric crisis.

45. Correct answer - 4. These are typical of oculogyric crisis. Option 1 is caused by shortening of the muscles on one side of the neck, drawing the head to one side. Option 2 is rapid movement of the eyeball. Option 3 is a spasm in the body in which the head bends back, the body bows outward, and the heels bend backward.
    CN: Physiological integrity

46. A client on the inpatient mental health unit is very suspicious. He does not interact with the other clients and appears to be constantly on his guard. Which of these measures should be included in the client's care plan?
    1. Placing the client on a bland diet.
    2. Preventing the client from spending time alone in his room rather than with other people.
    3. Asking probing questions during one-to-one interactions with the client.
    4. Avoiding talking with others when the client can see but not hear the conversation.

46. Correct answer - 4. When a suspicious client sees other people talking, he can mistakenly assume that the people are talking about him ("ideas of reference"). Therefore, the nurse should avoid such situations, because they reinforce the client's suspicion. Option 1: There is no need to place the client on a bland diet. Option 2: Because suspicious people fear intrusion from others and question their motives, care must be taken to respect the client's right to privacy. Time alone should be worked into the client's daily schedule. Option 3: A suspicious client should be allowed to control the amount of self-revelation that takes place in the interactions with the nurse. A probing approach will only alienate the client.
CN: Psychosocial integrity

47. A female client is hospitalized because she is in the manic phase of a bipolar disorder. The client is getting lithium carbonate (Eskalith). To determine if she is having an adverse reaction to Eskalith, which of these questions should the nurse consider?
    1. Is the client drooling?
    2. Is the client having any diarrhea?
    3. Is the client's blood pressure elevated?
    4. Is there blood in the client's urine?

47. Correct answer - 2. Adverse effects from lithium therapy include diarrhea, nausea, hair thinning, polydipsia, polyuria, edema, weight gain, mild hypoglycemia. Option 1, 3 and 4 are not adverse effects of lithium therapy.
CN: Psychosocial integrity

48. A client keeps touching the nurse on the arm and shoulder during their scheduled time together. The male nurse is uncomfortable with the client's touching. What would be the *best* way for the nurse to *initially* stop the client's touching behaviors?
    1. Tell the client to stop touching him.
    2. Limit the touching behavior to three times per visit.
    3. Tell the client her behavior is offensive and immature.
    4. Ask the client the meaning of the behavior.

48. Correct answer - 1. This sets a clear limit. Option 2 lets the touching continue. Option 3 is demeaning. Option 4 does not set a clear limit. It is a good second response, not an *initial* response.
CN: Psychosocial integrity

49. A neighbor tells you that she feels like a failure and sees nothing positive about her future. She says she has a barbiturate prescription in her purse and will fill it before the evening is over. The best action for you to take at this point would be to
    1. try to get your neighbor to see her positive points.
    2. point out all the things she has to live for (job, friends).
    3. get her to let you take her to the mental health center.
    4. tell her you will not stay with her unless she gives you the prescription.

49. Correct answer - 3. She is conveying suicide ideation. You are not the neighbor's nurse, and she needs professional help now. Take her to a place where she can get the help she needs. Options 1 and 2 do not address the neighbor's safety needs. Option 4 would not address the need for her safety. Even if she gave you the prescription, she would still be suicidal.
CN: Safe, effective care environment

50. A male client who is diagnosed as having schizophrenia, is admitted to the hospital. The client frequently assumes a fixed posture for about 4 hours at a time. Prior to planning care for this client, which of these questions is *essential* for the nurse to consider?
    1. Is the client married?
    2. Will the client be able to bathe himself?
    3. How can the client be provided with a diet that is high in calcium?
    4. Can a urine specimen be obtained to check for kidney stones?

50. Correct answer - 2. Clients who assume a fixed position for long periods frequently are unable to care for themselves and need assistance with ADLs. Option 1 is not essential in planning care. Options 3 and 4: The information provided does not indicate that the client requires a diet high in calcium or that the client is prone to develop kidney stones.
CN: Psychosocial integrity

51. A client who is depressed is to take amitriptyline (Elavil) and is taught the drug's adverse effects. Which of these statements, if made by the client, indicates that he understood the instructions?
    1. "I'm likely to have to urinate very frequently."
    2. "I'm likely to hear ringing in my ears."
    3. "I'm likely to get dizzy if I get up out of bed too quickly."
    4. "I'm likely to see halos around lights."

51. Correct answer - 3. Orthostatic hypotension is a adverse effect of the drug, so the client should change positions slowly to avoid dizziness. Options 1, 2, and 4 are not adverse effects of Elavil.
CN: Safe, effective care environment

52. At a staff meeting, the nurses are discussing a client who has refused to take his oral antipsychotic medication for 5 days. The client refuses the medication because it makes him feel "woozy-headed." The staff have noted that he isgetting more delusional and experiencing increased auditory hallucinations. Which of these comments by staff members offers the *best* approach in this situation?
    1. "We should disguise his medication by using the liquid form and giving it in juice."
    2. "We should inject his medication until he agrees to take it by mouth."
    3. "We should meet with him and outline a plan to restrict his privileges unless he takes his medication."
    4. "We should sit down with him and explore options to his current medication regimen."

53. Which symptoms would a nurse expect to assess in a client with schizophrenia?
    1. Distractibility, racing thoughts, psychomotor agitation
    2. Weight loss, sleep disturbance, problems with concentration
    3. Disorganized speech, disorganized behavior, delusions of grandeur
    4. Expansive or elevated mood, grandiosity, sleep disturbance

54. A 52-year-old woman was admitted 2 days ago to the inpatient psychiatric unit with a diagnosis of depression. This morning, after much urging and assistance, she bathed, dressed, and let the nurse fix her hair. A nurses aide exclaims, "Don't you look pretty! I guess you're feeling better now." The nurse speaks to the aide privately. Which statement, by the nurse to the aide, would be *most* appropriate?
    1. "Spend some time with the client today and try to cheer her up."
    2. "This client is still too depressed to be able to accept our compliments."
    3. "Making her look attractive has made her feel less depressed."
    4. "Try to get the client to put on some make-up."

52. Correct answer - 4. Staff must consider the client's right to refuse treatment and carefully review all treatment options with the client. Option 1 and 2: Disguising the medication in juice and giving the medication by injection against the client's will represent violations of his rights. Option 3: Restricting privileges in the absence of an agreed-upon contract is punitive.
CN: Safe, effective care environment

53. Correct answer - 3. This choice is the only one that lists the criteria for schizophrenia. Options 1, 2 and 4 are criteria for Bipolar I disorder, manic episode.
CN: Psychosocial integrity

54. Correct answer - 2. Premature compliments can increase depressive symptoms. Option 1: Attempts to "cheer up" the client will not be effective. Option 3: A client can look very attractive and still feel extremely depressed. Option 4: Applying make-up will not reduce this client's depression.
CN: Safe, effective care environment

55. A 48-year-old postal worker with a diagnosis of schizophrenia is admitted to the inpatient unit after making obscene remarks to his co-workers. He tells the nurse that he has always been a "loner" and has "heard voices for many years but they never interfered with my work in the mail room." Following the death of his mother 3 months ago, the voices have become angry and have been telling him to say "nasty things" to other people. Given this information, which of these statements would be a realistic short-term goal for this client?
    1. The client will no longer have auditory hallucinations.
    2. The client will have insight into his behavior.
    3. The client will return to work.
    4. The client will establish close personal friendships.

55. Correct answer - 3. A realistic short-term goal for this client is to return to work, where he had been functioning well. Option 1: It is unlikely that his auditory hallucinations will disappear. Option 2: Insight is not a priority since schizophrenic clients have difficulty thinking abstractly. Option 4: Because the client has a problem with basic trust, it is unlikely that he will develop close personal friendships.
CN: Psychosocial integrity

56. A 22-year-old client is admitted to the inpatient unit dressed in military fatigues. He salutes the charge nurse and asks, "Are you in charge of this prisoner-of-war camp? All you'll get out of me is my name, rank, and serial number." Which of these responses by the nurse would be *most* appropriate?
    1. "Why do you think that this is a prisoner-of-war camp?"
    2. "I am the charge nurse on this hospital unit."
    3. "You are a client on a psychiatric unit."
    4. "What are your name, rank, and serial number?

56. Correct answer - 2. The most appropriate response is a matter-of-fact statement answering the client's question about the nurse's identity and role. Option 1: Questions that ask "why" tend to make the client feel defensive, because he probably does not know "why." Option 3 is threatening because it directly challenges the client's delusion. Option 4: This supports and reinforces the client's delusion.
CN: Psychosocial integrity

57. The nurse assesses a client who is taking antipsychotic medication for signs of tardive dyskinesia, which include
    1. facial grimaces, worm-like movements of the tongue, and choreiform movements of the limbs.
    2. opisthotonos, oculogyric crisis, and muscle contractions of the neck.
    3. restlessness, leg aches, and shifting weight from foot to foot.
    4. akinesia, masklike facies, and small-stepped gait.

57. Correct answer - 1. Signs of tardive dyskinesia include facial grimaces, worm-like movements of the tongue, and choreiform movements of the limbs. Option 2 lists signs of a dystonic reaction. Option 3 lists signs of akathisia. Option 4 lists signs of Parkinsonian syndrome. All of these are possible adverse effects of antipsychotic medication.
CN: Physiological integrity

58. A client is diagnosed with dependent personality disorder. She asks the nurse if it's okay for her to call her children. What would be the best response for the nurse to make?
    1. "That's your decision."
    2. "What do you need to call them for?"
    3. "Why don't you wait since you'll be seeing them tomorrow."
    4. "I think that's a good idea."

58. Correct answer - 1. This option forces her to be assertive and decide for herself what to do. Option 2 is confrontational. Options 3 and 4 make the decision the nurse's, not the client's.
CN: Psychosocial integrity

59. One of the etiological theories of schizophrenia is a biochemical origin. Which neurochemical imbalance is most associated with schizophrenia?
    1. Serotonin
    2. Acetylcholine
    3. Norepinephrine
    4. Dopamine

59. Correct answer - 4. Dopamine causes overactive neural activity. Decreasing dopamine levels relieves psychotic symptoms. Option 1: Low serotonin is associated with depression. Option 2 is a neurochemical associated with Alzheimer's disease. Option 3: High levels of norepinephrine are associated with bipolar disorders, manic phase.
CN: Physiological integrity

60. A 35-year-old man comes to the Crisis Counseling Center following the abrupt break-up of his 10-year marriage. He states, "She left me for another man. I can't think straight. I can't manage this myself. Can you help me?" Recognizing that the client is in crisis, the nurse should *first* assist him to
   1. identify alternative solutions to the problem.
   2. explore earlier life experiences that sensitized him to this situation.
   3. attain an understanding of the precipitating event's effect on him.
   4. learn new, more effective coping methods to handle stress.

60. Correct answer - 3. The first task in crisis intervention is to clarify the precipitating event and the meaning of the event to the client. Options 1 and 4: Identifying alternative solutions and helping him to learn new coping methods would be done later. Option 2: The focus of crisis intervention is on the "here and now," rather than on exploring the psychodynamic origins of behavior.
CN: Psychosocial integrity

61. A client who has schizophrenia refuses her antipsychotic medication. What would be the best *first* action for the nurse to take?
   1. Honor the refusal and re-approach at a later time.
   2. Calmly state she needs the medication and ask why she is refusing.
   3. Tell the client she will lose privileges if she refuses.
   4. Ask the client why she thinks she doesn't need the medication.

61. Correct answer - 2. This is the best *first* action. It gives the client feedback and asks her to clarify her refusal. Option 1 would disrupt the dosing schedule and reinforce the negative behavior. Option 3 is illegal. Option 4: The client's thought processes are disorganized and, most likely, she would not be able to respond appropriately.
CN: Psychosocial integrity

62. A paranoid client paces the unit constantly and picks fights with other clients, accusing them of trying to harm him and prying into his private affairs. What is a priority nursing diagnosis for this client?
   1. Panic level anxiety related to being out of contact with reality.
   2. Fear related to accusing others of trying to harm him.
   3. Impaired social interaction related to picking fights with peers.
   4. Potential for other directed violence related to misinterpretation of environmental cues.

62. Correct answer - 4. The client's paranoid ideation and his aggressive behavior make this nursing diagnosis the priority because of his potential for harming others. Options 1, 2, and 3: The related to statements in these options are evidence of behaviors, not causes.
CN: Psychosocial integrity

63. Seclusion may be appropriate during a manic episode when the client
    1. engages in frantic, aimless physical activity.
    2. shouts loudly and continuously.
    3. shows extreme excitement when discussing something.
    4. plays the radio loudly.

63. Correct answer - 1. A manic client who is engaged in frantic, aimless physical activity is at risk for self-injury. Such clients have poor judgment and are impulsive; they can exhaust themselves physically if not controlled. Options 2, 3, and 4 would not lead to physical exhaustion and pose no risk to the client.
CN: Safe, effective care environment

64. A client is participating in a craft therapy session when she suddenly begins to shout at another client, "Stop watching me. I know what you're up to. I'll get you...." What would be the *best immediate* action for the nurse to take?
    1. Disband the group immediately.
    2. Instruct the client to follow the nurse to her room.
    3. Calmly tell the client that no one is watching her.
    4. Ask the other clients to stop looking at this person.

64. Correct answer - 2. The client needs to be removed from this environment and engaged in a concrete activity. If left in this situation, she could become violent. Option 1 would punish the others in the group. Option 3 ignores the client's fear. Option 4 would not address the client's problem and likely lead to physical aggression.
CN: Psychosocial integrity

65. A psychiatric client tells the nurse that the size of her nose is entirely too big and makes her ugly. The client demands referral to a plastic surgeon, saying a new nose will improve her life. What is the most likely diagnosis for this client?
    1. Somatization disorder
    2. Munchausen syndrome
    3. Body dysmorphic disorder
    4. Hypochondriasis

65. Correct answer - 3. The symptoms are classic for body dysmorphic disorder. Option 1 is characterized by many physical complaints. Option 2 is characterized by making oneself ill in order to receive needless treatment. Option 4 is characterized by a morbid fear of having a serious illness with no basis in fact.
CN: Psychosocial integrity

66. A client tells the nurse that nobody understands her. What would be the best *initial* reply for the nurse to make?
    1. "That's not true. I understand you."
    2. "You must be feeling awfully lonely."
    3. "How does it feel to not be understood?"
    4. "What is it that no one understands?"

66. Correct answer - 4. This is the only one that lets the nurse collect more information about what the client needs or is seeking. Options 1, 2, and 3 do not allow for obtaining needed information.
CN: Psychosocial integrity

67. A woman enters the emergency department carrying a limp 8-month-old baby. She calmly explains the baby quit breathing and she had a neighbor drive her to the hospital while she administered artificial respirations. The baby is revived. The nurse learns that this is the tenth emergency department visit for this mother and baby within the last 5 months. Which of the following should the nurse begin to suspect?
    1. Hyaline membrane disease
    2. A severe allergy in the child
    3. Munchausen by proxy syndrome
    4. Failure to thrive syndrome

67. Correct answer - 3. The mother's behavior combined with the frequency of emergency visits are typical of this syndrome. Option 1: Hyaline membrane disease occurs within hours of birth. Option 2: While it is possible this child could have severe allergies, the mother's calm behavior is typical of Munchausen by proxy syndrome. Option 4: Failure to thrive children lose weight and fail to grow.
CN: Psychosocial integrity

68. You are employed in an extended care facility. One of your elderly clients is to get Thorazine (chlorpromazine) 50 mg prn for agitation. What should you keep in mind when giving this drug?
    1. This medication has severe anticholinergic effects.
    2. Long-term use of this medication results in agranulocytosis.
    3. Cogentin should be administered prophylactically with this medication.
    4. Doing the AIMS test weekly can prevent adverse effects.

68. Correct answer - 1. Thorazine is not recommended for use in older adults because of anticholinergic effects. Options 2 and 3 are incorrect statements. Option 4: The AIMS test is used to *detect* tardive dyskinesia, *not* to prevent it.
CN: Physiological integrity

69. The *best* intervention to use with persons who have panic attacks is to
    1. teach the person how to recognize any triggers.
    2. have the person engage in aerobic exercise three times a week.
    3. teach the person how to identify cognitive errors.
    4. instruct the person to carry cue cards to use when having a panic attack.

69. Correct answer - 1. Knowing activities that trigger attacks gives the person the ability to avoid the triggers. Option 2: Aerobic exercise and excessive use of caffeine have been positively associated with panic attacks. Option 3: Cognitive errors have nothing to do with panic attacks. Option 4 is effective for people with O/CD, but would be ineffective during a panic attack when the person cannot focus on anything.
CN: Psychosocial integrity

70. The nurse is doing an intake assessment on a client who is flamboyantly dressed, seductive and dramatic in presentation, and tells the nurse that no one understands her. She has a history of alcohol abuse and sexual promiscuity. She also says she cannot understand why her "best friends" keep dumping her. Which disorder does this behavior suggest?
    1. Antisocial personality disorder
    2. Borderline personality disorder
    3. Narcissistic personality disorder
    4. Histrionic personality disorder

70. Correct answer - 4. This disorder is characterized by a sexually seductive appearance, demanding attention and approval in an exaggerated way. Option 1 would be characterized by negative social behavior such as truancy, excessive fighting, lying or animal cruelty. Option 2 would be diagnostic of clients with mood instability, unstable relationships , and transient psychotic states. Option 3 would be ascribed to clients who have exaggerated self importance and fantasies of brilliance, power and success.
CN: Psychosocial integrity

71. One of the clients on the psychiatric unit is actively suicidal. His care plan should include
    1. constant monitoring by the nursing staff.
    2. placement in seclusion until no longer suicidal.
    3. loss of privileges unless he promises not to harm himself.
    4. attend off-unit therapies only with staff or family.

71. Correct answer - 1. An actively suicidal person should not be left alone. Option 2: Placing the person in seclusion engenders feelings of abandonment and increases hopelessness. It is also punitive. Option 3 is punitive. Option 4 is not safe for the client who could "bolt."
CN: Safe, effective care environment

72. An elderly man enters the community mental health agency and tells you that he can't stand his son-in-law's attitude toward his daughter and he wants to know how he can get the son-in-law to change. What would be the best *initial* response for you to make?
    1. "Tell me about your daughter and son-in-law."
    2. "Before we talk about your son-in-law, let's talk about what prompted you to seek help."
    3. "Do you think you could get your daughter and her husband to come here with you?"
    4. "Sounds as if your son-in-law could be abusive."

72. Correct answer - 2. This lets the nurse collect more information about this man's needs. Options 1, 3, and 4 are not *initial* responses.
CN: Psychosocial integrity

73. A nurse is working with a client who says she is "very uptight" and has something to "get off her chest," but the nurse must promise to tell no one. What would be the *best* response for the nurse to make?
    1. "Is there a reason you have told no one before now?"
    2. "This sounds important. I'd like to hear what it is."
    3. "I will pass along, to other health-team members, what you tell me, if I feel the need."
    4. "How did you choose me as the person with whom to share this information?

73. Correct answer - 3. This is the *best* response and uses the principle of not keeping secrets. Option 1 puts the client on the defensive. Option 2 sounds good, but begs the issue of the "secret." Option 4: Who the client selected to share the secret with is irrelevant to the need to "get something off her chest."
CN: Psychosocial integrity

74. A client tells his nurse that his family would be happy if he left them. The nurse attended a family therapy session and has a very different perception of this client's family. How can the nurse help this client get a more objective grasp of his standing in his family?
    1. Express disagreement with his perception and why.
    2. Ask him how he knows his family wants him to leave.
    3. Ask him how it feels to be an outsider in his own family.
    4. Have him write his family a letter expressing his feelings.

74. Correct answer - 2. This choice is the only one that invites the client to examine what happened in his family session and how he erroneously arrived at the conclusion that his family wanted him to leave them. Options 1, 3, and 4 are therefore not correct.
CN: Psychosocial integrity

75. The home health care nurse arrives at a client's residence about 30 minutes late. The client greets the nurse with a barrage of profanities and tells the nurse not to ever keep him waiting again. What is the *best* way for the nurse to respond?
    1. State she will not stay if he continues to be verbally abusive.
    2. Explain why she was unavoidably detained and apologize profusely.
    3. Express concern that this outburst indicates poor coping on his part.
    4. Apologize for the lateness and comment about the intensity of his feelings.

75. Correct answer - 4. The client's response is excessively inappropriate for the nurse' lateness. The intensity indicates something else is going on that has nothing to do with her lateness. Option 1 is threatening. Option 2 would demean the nurse herself. Option 3 may be true but it is not the best way to respond at this time.
CN: Psychosocial integrity

76. A young man who has just learned he is HIV positive calls *Ask-A-Nurse* and asks, in a trembling voice, "Am I going to die? I just found out I am HIV positive." What would be the best *initial* response for the nurse to make?
    1. "It is highly unlikely you will die soon."
    2. "How did you come to the conclusion you were dying?"
    3. "What does knowing you will soon die mean to you?"
    4. "I'm not sure how to answer that question."

77. Setting limits would be most appropriate when the manic client
    1. engages in frenetic aimless physical activity.
    2. repeatedly changes the TV in the activity room without asking.
    3. frequently questions staff about mealtimes.
    4. asks for help with using the telephone.

78. A nurse has an African American client who gives her only fleeting eye contact. What is the best way, *initially,* for the nurse to assess the meaning of the client's behavior?
    1. Ask the client directly what his behavior means.
    2. Consult with an authority on African-American behavior.
    3. Ask an African-American colleague about the meaning of the behavior.
    4. Attend a cultural diversity class to learn about culture-specific behaviors.

76. Correct answer - 2. This is the only option that lets the nurse gather further information about the caller's needs. Options 1, 3, and 4 all preclude the client's providing more information.
CN: Psychosocial integrity

77. Correct answer - 2. Clients in the manic phase of bipolar disorder may have trouble distinguishing boundaries and frequently intrude on the space of others. Such a situation may become volatile if the other clients become annoyed and voice irritation to the client. Option 1 requires structure for safety. Option 3 is anxious behavior. Option 4 is a processing issue, not a limit setting one.
CN: Psychosocial integrity

78. Correct answer - 1. The best first action to take is to ask directly. Options 2, 3, and 4 are good *secondary* actions.
CN: Psychosocial integrity

79. A male client tells you that his wife's nagging really gets on his nerves. He asks you if you will talk with her about it during their next family session. The most therapeutic response for you to make would be
    1. "Tell me more specifically about her complaints."
    2. "Can you think why she might nag you so much?"
    3. "I'll help you think about how to bring this up yourself."
    4. "Why do you want me to initiate this rather than you?"

79. Correct answer - 3. The client needs to learn how to communicate directly with his wife about her behavior. Helping him to do this will let him to practice a new skill, as well as communicate your confidence in his ability to directly confront this situation. Options 1 and 2 direct attention away from the client and place attention inappropriately on his wife, who is not there. Option 4 implies that there might be a legitimate reason for you to assume responsibility for something that rightfully belongs to the client. He will spend precious time convincing you why you should do his work.
CN: Psychosocial integrity

80. During a group session with six other clients, a female client tells you she's sure that another client is discussing group business with individuals who are not in the group. She says she is no longer willing to share anything with the group because of the other client's "big mouth." What is your *best* response?
    1. "I want you to tell the client to stop doing that."
    2. "How do you know the client has done this?"
    3. "I wouldn't share anything else in the group either."
    4. "How do you feel about what that person is doing?"

80. Correct answer - 2. This will assist the person to objectively examine facts rather than impressions. Options 1, 3, and 4: None of these help the client critically examine her perceptions to determine if her interpretation of the client's behavior is valid.
CN: Psychosocial integrity

81. Which of the following should the nurse be most concerned about when caring for a client taking an antianxiety medication?
    1. Dependence
    2. Transient hypertension
    3. Abrupt withdrawal
    4. Constipation

81. Correct answer - 3. Abrupt discontinuation of an antianxiety drug can lead to withdrawal symptoms. Antianxiety medications usually are prescribed for short periods. Option 1: If used over a prolonged period, such drugs may produce psychological or physical dependence. Options 2 and 4 are not associated with antianxiety drugs.
CN: Physiological integrity

82. A client tells her therapy group that she has started practicing conscious relaxation. She is pleased with its effectiveness in reducing her need to wash her hands. One group member responds by saying that conscious relaxation is a bunch of nonsense. As group leader, what is the nurse's *best* intervention?
    1. Ask the group member why he feels the need to discount the client's experience.
    2. Ask the group member why he thinks the technique worked so well for this client.
    3. Foster group cohesiveness by asking the member to keep negative opinions to himself.
    4. Ask the member to share his understanding and experience with conscious relaxation.

82. Correct answer - 4. This response seeks to clarify the group member's experience and provide the opportunity for the group leader or any other member to further explain the purpose of conscious relaxation. Option 1 makes the issue a personal one and may feel accusatory. Option 2 takes the focus away from the client's concern. Option 3 does not foster group cohesiveness and conveys disapproval of negative statements.
CN: Psychosocial integrity

83. A nurse is the leader of a therapy group. At the first session, one group member accuses the nurse of being far too pushy and says the nurse does not have the right to pressure anyone. Which response would *best* help the client remain non-defensive?
    1. "I sense that you are not comfortable in the group."
    2. "Thank you for the feedback. I'll work on being less pushy."
    3. "Sounds as if the group is stimulating some of your issues."
    4. "Tell me about one time when you felt pushed or pressured."

83. Correct answer - 4. This gives specific examples, which helps the client become more objective. Option 1 may feel accusatory and raise the client's defensiveness. Option 2 does not permit exploration of the client's statement. Option 3 is too direct a statement during the early stage of group work and will increase client's defensiveness.
CN: Psychosocial integrity

84. When planning the care of a client with GAD, which intervention is most important to include?
    1. Encourage the client to engage in activities that increase feelings of power and self-esteem.
    2. Promote the client's interaction and socialization with others.
    3. Help the client make plans for regular periods of leisure time.
    4. Encourage the client to use a diary to record when anxiety occurred, its causes, and which interventions may have helped.

84. Correct answer - 4. One of the nurse's goals is to help the client to associate symptoms with an event, thereby beginning to learn appropriate ways to eliminate or reduce distress. A diary can be a beneficial tool for this purpose. Options 1, 2, and 3 may be appropriate for this client, but they are not the priority.
CN: Psychosocial integrity

HOW TO SCORE AND USE THE DIAGNOSTIC PROFILE

In the top "QUESTION NUMBER" row of boxes, mark each question number you answered wrong. Under each question number, check the box in the "TEST TAKING SKILLS" section that is the most appropriate reason you answered the question incorrectly. Do the same for the "CLIENT NEED CATEGORIES" section. The client need category code follows the rationale. Total the number of check marks, by line, in the "Totals" column. This provides you with a profile of your weak areas that should be improve upon prior to taking the NCLEX-RN.

PERSONAL DIAGNOSTIC PROFILE

QUESTION NUMBER																						Totals

TEST-TAKING SKILLS

Misread the question																						
Missed important point																						
Forgot fact or concept																						
Applied wrong fact or concept																						
Drew wrong conclusion																						
Incorrectly evaluated distractors																						
Mistakenly selected answer choice																						
Read into the question																						
Made a wrong guess																						
Misunderstood question																						

CLIENT NEED CATEGORIES

Safe, effective care environment																						
Physiological integrity																						
Psychosocial integrity																						
Health promotion and maintenance																						

CALCULATING SUBSCORES

After you score your test, determine your subscores in these client need categories by filling in the following grid.

CLIENT NEED

	Safe, effective care environment	Physiological integrity	Psychosocial integrity	Health promotion & maintenance
Number of questions	17	12	55	0
Number incorrect				
Number correct				
Percent correct*				

*To determine the percent correct in each category, divide the number of items answered correctly by the total number of items and multiply the result by 100.

Note: This is a short test with a limited sample of items in each category. Therefore, if a score in any category is less than 75% correct, further study is strongly advised.

CHAPTER 4

TAKING THIS SKILL TEST

Your Study Guide Module has instructed you to take the following skill test after you have completed your review of the clinical area. This test will give you needed experience in answering NCLEX-RN type questions and will give you a good idea of your competence in this clinical area.

The format of the skill test gives you instant feedback as you take it. Each question is in the left column. The correct answer with rationale is in the right column.

As you read each question in the lefthand column, cover the righthand column with an index card until you have selected your answer. Slide the card down, keeping remaining question answers covered. When you have completed the test, use the Personal Diagnostic Profile to record why you answered any question incorrectly.

If you scored lower than 75% on this skill test, you should analyze the reason and go back and do further review. You may also wish to consult a current nursing textbook for any areas that are unclear to you.

1. A newborn with esophageal atresia is to have a repair. Which postoperative nursing measure should be implemented *first?*
   1. Place him in a prone position, with his head slightly elevated and turned to the side.
   2. Place him in a side-lying position, with his neck hyperextended.
   3. Give the first oral feeding with sterile water 24 hours after surgery.
   4. Change his position every 2 hours from his back to his side, keeping the head slightly elevated.

1. Correct answer - 4. The head is elevated to facilitate drainage of secretions. The position is changed frequently to maintain skin integrity and to prevent pneumonia. Option 1: The prone position compresses the abdomen and may cause gastric reflux. Option 2: Hyperextension of the neck puts pressure on the suture line of the esophagus. Option 3: Oral feedings are not started until 2 to 10 days after surgery.
CN: Physiological integrity

2. A 2-year-old girl returns from surgery with a temporary colostomy after a bowel resection for Hirschsprung's disease. Which immediate postoperative nursing intervention for the client would have priority?
   1. Change the surgical dressing.
   2. Suction the nasopharynx frequently to remove secretions.
   3. Irrigate the colostomy with 100 ml of normal saline solution.
   4. Auscultate her breath sounds.

2. Correct answer - 4. The immediate nursing intervention after surgery would be to assess pulmonary function. Option 1: Tthe surgical dressing should not require changing right away. Option 2: Suctioning should be performed only if the client cannot maintain a patent airway. Option 3: Colostomy irrigation is not warranted.
CN: Physiological integrity

3. A 2-week-old boy has returned from surgery for correction of pyloric stenosis. Which postoperative nursing management would be most important?
   1. Feed as tolerated, assess the amount of emesis, and encourage parental involvement in care.
   2. Give the infant nothing by mouth until the wound heals and encourage parental involvement.
   3. Monitor intake and output (I&O), and encourage parental involvement in care.
   4. Monitor hydration status and encourage parental involvement.

3. Correct answer - 1. Feedings are resumed gradually after surgery. Occasional emesis is common after surgery, and nurses need to let parents know about this. Parental involvement is a must, both pre- and postoperatively, to promote bonding and decrease feelings of guilt. Option 2: There is no reason to restrict oral feeding. Options 3 and 4: Assessing and developing feeding tolerance are of primary importance.
CN: Physiological integrity

4. A 4-year-old boy with acute lymphocytic leukemia has been receiving vincristine. Which sign would be most important for the nurse to evaluate during vincristine therapy?
   1. Diarrhea
   2. Hematuria
   3. Moon face and fluid retention
   4. Weakness and constipation

4. Correct answer - 4. Vincristine is a plant alkaloid. Neurotoxicity is a possible adverse effect of vincristine therapy and may be manifested as weakness and constipation. Option 1: Peristalsis is reduced, not increased, with vincristine. Option 2: Hematuria is an adverse effect of Cytoxan (cyclophosphamide). Option 3: Moon face and fluid retention are adverse effects of prednisone.
CN: Physiological integrity

5. A 4-year-old girl is admitted to the hospital with suspected leukemia. Which of the following would be the best room assignment?
   1. With a 4-year-old girl who has rheumatoid arthritis.
   2. Alone in a private room.
   3. With a 4-year-old girl who has leukemia.
   4. With a 5-year-old boy who is having a tonsillectomy.

5. Correct answer - 2. Avoiding exposure to infection requires a private room. Options 1, 3, and 4: Cross-infection could occur from being with any of these children.
CN: Physiological integrity

6. A 2-year-old girl has been successfully treated for croup. Her parents ask, "What should we do if she gets croup again?" What is the nurse's best response?
   1. "You don't have to worry. She now has immunity to croup and will not get it again."
   2. "Come to the emergency department immediately when she starts coughing."
   3. "If she gets another cold, watch for croup. Keep a cool-mist humidifier running in her room, and give her lots of liquids."
   4. "You could put a crib in the bathroom and let her sleep with the hot shower running to make steam."

6. Correct answer - 3. A child can get croup again, particularly during an upper respiratory infection. The symptoms of croup may be relieved or lessened through adequate hydration and increased humidity. Option 1: An attack of coup does not confer immunity. Option 2: This may cause unnecessary parental anxiety and dependency on the health care provider; it does not teach how to control croup. Option 4: This is unsafe; a child should never be left alone in the bathroom with hot water running.
CN: Health promotion and maintenance

7. Which is the most significant finding in a history related to developmental hip dysplasia?
   1. The mother's third trimester activity.
   2. Breech presentation at birth.
   3. The client's serum calcium level at birth.
   4. An Apgar score of 6 at 5 minutes.

7. Correct answer - 2. Breech presentation is a factor frequently associated with developmental hip dysplasia. Options 1, 3, and 4 have no bearing on hip dysplasia.
CN: Physiological integrity

8. When a 1-year-old client returns from a cardiac catheterization, the nurse notes that the pulse distal to the catheter insertion site is weaker. What is the *first* action the nurse should take?
   1. Remove the pressure bandage from the insertion site.
   2. Perform passive exercises on the affected extremity.
   3. Notify the health care provider of the assessment.
   4. Record the data on the nursing notes.

8. Correct answer - 4. The pulse distal to the insertion site may be weaker for a few hours but should gradually increase in strength. Option 1: The pressure dressing should not be removed because of the risk of hemorrhage. Option 2: Such exercises would not be performed after a cardiac catheterization. Option 3: The health care provider does not need to be notified at this time.
CN: Physiological integrity

9. A 12-month-old girl is at the clinic for a well-baby checkup. During the examination, the nurse discovers that her teeth are full of caries and that she still uses a bottle. What is the nurse's *best* intervention?
   1. Ask her mother about her knowledge of dental caries and bottle weaning.
   2. Tell the mother that dental caries are caused by leaving the baby sleep with a bottle full of milk.
   3. Ask the mother about the client's bedtime routine.
   4. Tell the mother to stop the bottle and to see a dentist right away.

9. Correct answer - 3. This open-ended question lets the nurse gather information without attaching blame. Option 1: Asking the mother about her knowledge is likely to put her on the defensive. Option 2: This response is quick to assign blame. Option 4: The tone of this response is inappropriately peremptory.
CN: Health promotion and maintenance

10. What is the *best* activity for an 11-year-old girl in sickle-cell crisis?
    1. Bowling
    2. Playing with paper dolls
    3. Swimming
    4. Painting

10. Correct answer - 4. While a child is in sickle-cell crisis, oxygen consumption needs to be minimized. Of the options listed, painting is the only quiet and age-appropriate activity. Options 1 and 3 are too strenuous for a child in sickle-cell crisis. Option 2 is not an age-appropriate activity for an 11-year-old girl.
CN: Physiological integrity

11. A boy born with a complete cleft palate and unilateral cleft lip has just returned from the recovery room after a surgical repair of the defect. His vital signs are stable and he is awake and active. What is the nurse's *initial* intervention?
    1. Restrain his elbows.
    2. Position him on his abdomen.
    3. Take his vital signs.
    4. Provide pain medication.

11. Correct answer - 1. Because the infant is awake and active, the suture area must be protected. Option 2: The client should not be positioned on his abdomen, as this can cause trauma to the suture line. Option 3: Although vital signs are important, the recovery room nurse reported that they were stable; therefore, the restraints are more important at this time. Option 4: Pain medication may be required soon, but vital signs should be reassessed before it is administered.
CN: Physiological integrity

12. A 5-month-old girl has had recurrent middle-ear infections since she was 3 months old. What is *most* important to assess when she comes for a visit?
    1. How well she eats
    2. Her weight gain since her last visit
    3. Her taking all the prescribed antibiotics for the last infection
    4. Her temperature

13. The mother of a 3-year-old boy calls the hospital sobbing that he has swallowed some Tylenol. What should the nurse learn *first?*
    1. How the child gained access to the Tylenol.
    2. The number and strength of the Tylenol ingested.
    3. Whether the child looks jaundiced.
    4. Whether the child is complaining of right upper quadrant abdominal tenderness.

14. Which of the following should the nurse teach parents to help them prevent rheumatic fever in their child?
    1. Avoid exposing the child to streptococcal organisms.
    2. Insist that a sore throat in the child be treated with antibiotics.
    3. Learn the signs and symptoms of rheumatic fever.
    4. Report symptoms and cooperate with treatment of streptococcal infection.

15. A 6-year-old girl was treated 8 weeks ago for strep throat. She returns to the clinic with another sore throat and fever, and she now has a rash and complains of joint pain. She is admitted to the hospital with a diagnosis of rheumatic fever. Which strategy will *best* help prevent permanent damage?
    1. Promote early ambulation to reduce joint stiffness and pain.
    2. Maintain bed rest to reduce cardiac workload.
    3. Limit visitors and maintain a quiet room to minimize central nervous system stimulation.
    4. Avoid salicylates (aspirin) to avoid risk of Reye's syndrome.

12. Correct answer - 3. If the client is not receiving her full course of antibiotic therapy, her ear infections will recur; permanent hearing loss or systemic infection may result. Parents may not understand this and may discontinue treatment when the infant seems better. Options 1, 2, and 4 are important aspects to assess, but none is as critical as ensuring full cooperation with antibiotic therapy.
CN: Physiological integrity

13. Correct answer - 2. Initial assessment requires finding out how much Tylenol the child has ingested to determine whether the amount is toxic for height and weight. Option 1: Safety measures should be taught after the emergency is resolved. Option 3: Jaundice would be a late sign of liver toxicity. Option 4: Right upper quadrant tenderness indicates liver toxicity, which would occur 1 or more days after ingesting a toxic amount of Tylenol.
CN: Physiological integrity

14. Correct answer - 4. Prevention or treatment of group A streptococcal infection prevents rheumatic fever. Option 1: This is not realistic; it is usually impossible to know when one is being exposed. Option 2: This would be an inappropriate use of antibiotics; many sore throats are viral and would not respond to antibiotic treatment. Option 3: This option does not prevent the occurrence of rheumatic fever.
CN: Health promotion and maintenance

15. Correct answer - 2. The prognosis for rheumatic fever depends on the extent of myocardial involvement. Activity must be limited until cardiac status is normal. Option 1: There are not permanent after-effects of joint involvement. Option 3: There are no permanent after-effects of chorea. Option 4: Salicylates (aspirin) are prescribed for pain and fever accompanying rheumatic fever, which is associated with antibodies to streptococcal bacteria. Reye's syndrome is associated with the use of aspirin for viral infections.
CN: Physiological integrity

16. The teacher of a 6-year-old boy who had rheumatic fever 3 months ago tells the school nurse that he is not paying attention in school. Which intervention would be *most* important for the nurse to make?
    1. Observe his social interactions with other children in the class.
    2. Keep him away from children who sneeze or cough.
    3. Watch him for clumsiness or other neurologically based changes.
    4. Test him frequently to ensure that he has kept up with his schoolwork.

16. Correct answer - 3. Sydenham's chorea, a common sequel to rheumatic fever, is commonly manifested by clumsiness, irritability, and other neurologic changes. It can occur from several weeks to several months after the initial bout of rheumatic fever. Option 1: Nothing in the case study indicates that the client is having a problem with social interactions. Option 2: This is nearly impossible to accomplish and does not address the problem. Option 4: This would put undue pressure on the client.
    CN: Physiological integrity

17. A 3-year-old boy has nephrotic syndrome. Which would be the *best* nursing goal for him?
    1. Provide analgesia, maintain fluid restriction, and promote adequate rest.
    2. Provide rest, maintain skin integrity, and promote adequate nutritional intake.
    3. Provide vigorous diverse activities, and promote adequate nutritional intake.
    4. Promote bed rest, maintain fluid restriction, and provide analgesia.

17. Correct answer - 2. Children with nephrotic syndrome are commonly lethargic and need to conserve energy. Edema requires careful attention to skin care, and anorexia requires attention to adequate nutritional intake. Options 1 and 4: Analgesia is not needed in nephrotic syndrome. Option 3: Vigorous activities are not recommended for a child with nephrotic syndrome.
    CN: Physiological integrity

18. What is the *best* teaching point for a client with type 1 diabetes?
    1. Advise that insulin be stored in a cool place.
    2. Encourage the client to rotate injection sites daily from thigh to abdomen to arm.
    3. Emphasize that the insulin vial be shaken vigorously to mix the medication.
    4. Advise that the short-acting insulin be drawn up last when two insulins are mixed.

18. Correct answer - 1. Insulin should be stored in a cool place so that the protein potency is not altered. Option 2: The client should use one area (for example, the arm) for about a week, then rotate to another area, not change daily. Option 3: Insulin vials should be gently rolled to minimize the number of air bubbles created in a vial. Option 4: Short-acting insulin should be drawn up first so as not to contaminate the vial with longer-acting insulin.
    CN: Safe, effective care environment

19. Which of the following would *best* ensure responsible insulin administration by a 9-year-old boy?
    1. He observes his parents as they administer his injection.
    2. He learns to draw up his insulin but does not inject it.
    3. He learns to administer his insulin with supervision.
    4. He manages his insulin administration independently.

19. Correct answer - 3. School-age children can administer their own insulin, but supervision is needed to ensure correct procedure and dosage. Options 1 and 2 give the client too little responsibility. Option 4 gives him too much responsibility.
    CN: Health promotion and maintenance

20. Which statement by an 8-year-old girl with diabetes mellitus indicates that she understands glycosylated hemoglobin assessment?
    1. "The test will be inaccurate if I ate candy yesterday."
    2. "The test replaces home blood glucose monitoring."
    3. "The test assesses a type of anemia acquired by people with insulin-dependent diabetes."
    4. "The test gives an average blood glucose level for the past 3 months."

20. Correct answer - 4. Glycosylated hemoglobin assessment measures red blood cells with glucose molecules attached. Because life span of a red blood cell is about 3 months and the glucose remains attached until the cell dies, the test is an average of the blood glucose level over 3 months. Option 1: One day's intake does not determine the test result. Option 2: The goal of the test is to assess long-term control, not to determine the blood glucose level at one point in time. Option 3: The test is not for anemia.
CN: Health promotion and maintenance.

21. Which eating plan would be *most* effective for a 3-year-old boy with nephrotic syndrome?
    1. Let him eat when he feels like it because of his developmental age.
    2. Give him small, frequent meals high in carbohydrates and fat.
    3. Give him small, frequent meals and liquids or high-protein milk shakes.
    4. Keep his mealtimes the same to decrease his anxiety over his illness.

21. Correct answer - 3. A child with nephrotic syndrome is often lethargic and anorexic. Small nourishing meals will be the most beneficial. Option 1: His developmental age has nothing to do with his anorexia. Option 2: A high-fat meal would exacerbate his hyperlipidemia. Option 4: He is not anxious but rather anorexic.
CN: Physiological integrity

22. A 9-month-old infant has acute bronchiolitis. Ribavirin is ordered three times a day, using a small particle aerosol generator. Which outcome would *best* indicate that this medication has produced its desired effect?
    1. Barrel chest is less evident.
    2. Secretions are liquified.
    3. Coughing episodes increase.
    4. Wheezing is diminished.

22. Correct answer - 1. Ribavirin is an antiviral agent that prohibits replication of respiratory syncytial virus (RSV), which is the most common cause of bronchiolitis. The hyper-inflated or barrel chest is a classic sign of bronchiolitis and is caused by obstruction in the small air passages. The resolution of the virus results in decreased airway obstruction and less trapped air. Option 2: Ribavirin is not a mucolytic agent. Option 3: Paroxysms of coughing occur with bronchiolitis. Resolution of the disease process decreases frequency, not increase occurrence. Option 4: Ribavirin is not a bronchodilator.
CN: Physiological integrity

23. A female infant with acute bronchiolitis is on the pediatric unit with an NPO order. The mother asks "Why can't she drink?" Which statement by the nurse *best* explains the reason for the NPO order?
    1. "She doesn't need as many calories now."
    2. "There is a very big possibility of fluid overload."
    3. "Feeding her now would be too much of an effort for her."
    4. "Her digestive system has slowed down because of the infection."

23. Correct answer - 3. Oral feedings during the acute phase of this illness will increase hypoxemia. The effort expended in feeding may result in tachypnea, weakness and fatigue. Intravenous feedings are preferred during the acute phase. Option 1: During the acute phase of this illness, her caloric need will actually increase because her basal metabolism will increase. Option 2: While hydration status must be continuously monitored by the nurse to assure adequate hydration and prevent pulmonary edema, this is not the primary reason why the child is NPO. Option 4: Increased peristalsis and acute diarrhea are often associated with infections outside the alimentary canal. The nurse should not expect peristalsis to decrease
CN: Physiological integrity

24. A 4½-year-old girl is to get digoxin 0.04 mg at 9 a.m. The nurse checks her apical pulse and notes that it is 82 beats per minute (bpm) and irregular. Which interpretation, by the nurse, would be the *most* correct?
    1. She just woke up and the pulse is slower in the morning.
    2. She may be experiencing digoxin toxicity.
    3. This is perfectly normal for a child of this age.
    4. She may be developing hypokalemia.

24. Correct answer - 4. The rate of 82 bpm would be generally considered within normal limits for a 4½-year-old child. An irregular rhythm is not normal and might indicate hypokalemia secondary to digoxin therapy. Her potassium level should be checked as soon as possible. Option 1: This is not an accurate statement. Option 2: Her pulse rate of 82 is *not* a sign of toxicity, although an irregular pulse may be. Option 3: An irregular pulse is not a normal finding.
CN: Physiological integrity

25. A 2-month-old girl with congestive heart failure, secondary to tetralogy of Fallot, has been admitted to the hospital. She has been digitalized and her condition is now stable. While making rounds, the nurse observes that she is crying, dyspneic, and her lips are cyanotic. In addition to starting ordered oxygen, the nurse should next place her
    1. in a supine, extended position.
    2. pacifier in her mouth.
    3. in a lateral, knee-chest position.
    4. in modified Trendelenburg's position.

25. Correct answer - 3. The child's respiratory efforts will be enhanced by placing her in a lateral, knee-chest position. Option 1: A supine position would not relieve the respiratory distress and could aggravate it. Option 2: The pacifier may interfere with the infant's need to mouth breathe. Option 4: Modified Trendelenburg's position would not relieve the respiratory distress and may aggravate it.
CN: Physiological integrity

26. A 6-year-old girl has just had a cardiac catheterization. The right femoral vein was used for the cutdown site. What is the *best* post-procedure position for this client?
    1. Right-side lying, with blanket roll between knees.
    2. On her back with right leg immobilized by sandbags.
    3. Semi-Fowler's position with knees slightly flexed.
    4. On her abdomen with feet over end of mattress.

27. The mother of a newborn who has hypospadias tells the nurse that since her baby looks okay and is able to urinate, she does not see a need for him to have corrective surgery. To properly teach the mother about the need for surgery, what is the nurse's *best* response?
    1. "His self-image and normal sexual function make the surgery necessary."
    2. "The surgery will help maintain proper fluid balance and nutrition."
    3. "Proper hormone levels and normal mobility require the surgery to done."
    4. "His sexual maturation and freedom from pain make the surgery necessary."

28. A 3-year-old boy has been returned to his room following surgery to correct hypospadias. In order to prevent separation of the incision, which action would be *best* for the nurse to take?
    1. Position him in a semi-Fowler's position.
    2. Elevate the scrotal sac on a folded sheepskin.
    3. Use restraints as needed to keep him from touching the area.
    4. Clean the area every 2 hours with diluted hydrogen peroxide.

26. Correct answer - 2. Immediately after a cardiac catheterization, she should be flat with extremities straight and immobilized to prevent an increase in intravascular pressure, which may cause bleeding. Options 1 and 3 would result in flexion of the leg at the cut-down site, increasing intravascular pressure which may cause bleeding. Option 4: This position prevents direct observation of pressure bandage.
CN: Physiological integrity

27. Correct answer - 1. Objectives of surgery are to enable the child to void in the normal standing position, improve appearance of the genitalia, and produce a sexually adequate organ. Options 2, 3, and 4 are not relevant to problems associated with hypospadias.
CN: Health promotion and maintenance

28. Correct answer - 2. Elevating the affected area on a Bellevue Bridge (or similar structure) will help prevent separation of the suture line as well as preventing dependent edema. Option 1 would increase the swelling. Option 3 is not specific to incision separation. Staying with him instead of restraining him would be more appropriate. Option 4 would have no effect on incision separation.
CN: Physiological integrity

29. The nurse is planning for the discharge of a 9-year-old boy with type 1diabetes. Which action indicates the client understands the correct techniques for drawing up regular and NPH insulin?
    1. He injected air first into the regular insulin vial and then into the NPH insulin vial. He then withdrew the NPH insulin followed by the regular insulin.
    2. He injected air first into the NPH insulin vial and then into the regular insulin vial. He then withdrew the regular insulin and then the NPH insulin.
    3. He mixed 5 syringes of both type of insulin and left them in the refrigerator for a week's use.
    4. He avoided mixing the different types of insulin in the same syringe.

29. Correct answer - 2. Longer-action insulin (NPH) binds with regular insulin. Regular should be withdrawn first to avoid contamination with longer-acting insulin. Option 1 is the incorrect order. Option 3: Insulin should be used within 5 minutes of mixing. Option 4 is wrong because different insulins can be mixed.
CN: Health promotion and maintenance

30. A12-year-old boy is seen in the clinic for suspected diabetes mellitus. Results of tests confirm the diagnosis, and he is placed on a daily regimen of isophane (NPH) insulin. Because he is to get NPH insulin every morning, what should he be taught to include in his daily care?
    1. Eating a mid-afternoon snack.
    2. Avoiding strenuous exercise.
    3. Limiting fluid intake after the evening meal.
    4. Scheduling periods of rest throughout the day.

30. Correct answer - 1. A person taking NPH insulin should be instructed that a mid-afternoon shack may be required, because mid-afternoon precedes the onset of the peak action of NPH insulin. Option 2: Taking NPH insulin does not preclude physical exercise. Option 3: There is no need to limit fluid intake after the evening meal. Option 4: Treatment with NPH insulin does not require scheduled periods of rest throughout the day.
CN: Physiological integrity

31. A teenage girl with scoliosis has halo-pelvic traction applied. What would be the most likely neurological sign of excessive traction?
    1. Upper and lower extremity hyporeflexia
    2. Pupil inequality with fixed dilation.
    3. Loss of lateral vision and inability to follow a moving object.
    4. Diminished peripheral pulses in the lower legs.

31. Correct answer - 3. These are classic signs of excessive traction. Option 1: Hyperreflexia, not hyporeflexia may be an early sign of neurologic damage. Option 2: Unequal pupils are a sign of advanced neurological damage. Option 4: Diminished pulses would suggest circulatory problems rather than neurological.
CN: Physiological integrity

32. A 14-month-old boy is admitted to the pediatric unit with a fractured right femur. He is placed in Bryant's (vertical) traction. His mother asks the nurse the purpose of the traction. The nurse's response should be based on the understanding that the primary purpose of the traction is to
    1. increase circulation to the affected bone.
    2. keep the bones in proper alignment.
    3. prevent edema.
    4. avoid the development of a fat embolism.

32. Correct answer - 2. The purpose of the traction is to reduce the fracture by bringing the ends of the broken bone into alignment. Option 1 may cause circulation to be obstructed. Option 3: The primary purpose is to place the bones in alignment, not to prevent swelling. Option 4: At the time a bone is fractured, fat globules may move into the circulation (although not commonly seen in children). Traction will not prevent an embolism.
CN: Physiological integrity

33. A pediatric client is to have a surgical repair of the pylorus. In preparation for surgery, the nurse administers a vitamin K injection to
    1. assist in wound healing.
    2. promote the return of peristaltic action.
    3. lessen the likelihood of nerve damage.
    4. decrease the possibility of postoperative bleeding.

33. Correct answer - 4. Vitamin K is essential for blood clotting. Option 1: Vitamin C is more likely to be given for this purpose, because vitamin K does not have this action. Option 2: Vitamin K does not cause peristaltic action, and peristaltic action is not a desirable outcome in the immediate postoperative period. Option 3: Vitamin K does not have this action.
CN Physiological integrity

34. The nurse can expect to find which of the following symptoms in a client with sickle-cell crisis?
    1. A macular-papular rash
    2. Loose stools
    3. Abdominal pain
    4. Hair loss

34. Correct answer - 3. The sickled RBCs occlude the capillaries in the mesentery, spleen and liver causing severe pain. Option 1: A rash is not a symptom related to sickle cell crisis or anemia. Option 2: Because the child generally vomits and may be dehydrated, diarrhea is not an expected symptom. Option 4: Hair loss is not an expected symptom.
CN: Physiological integrity

35. A client who had a pyloromyotomy is to be bottle fed for the first time. After the feeding, it is best for the nurse to position him
    1. with his head lower than his chest.
    2. with his head hyperextended.
    3. on his back.
    4. with his head elevated and his body turned on right side.

35. Correct answer - 4. This position prevents him from aspirating his vomitus. Option 1: Gravity should be use to aid in digestion of feeding. Option 2: This position is not comfortable or necessary. Option 3: Aspiration of vomitus is more likely to occur in this position.
CN: Safe, effective care environment

36. A 2-year-old girl's developmental level is within normal limits when she can
    1. run without falling.
    2. hop on one leg.
    3. button clothing.
    4. catch a ball.

36. Correct answer - 1. This is within developmental limits for a 2-year-old child. Options 2, 3, and 4 are expected behaviors of a 4-year-old child.
CN: Health promotion and maintenance

37. A 2-year-old boy is admitted to the hospital in acute respiratory distress. Cystic fibrosis (CF) is diagnosed. Which statement, made by his mother, would the nurse expect with a diagnosis of CF?
    1. "He has never had lung problems before."
    2. "He has a salty taste when I kiss him."
    3. "His stools are small and dry."
    4. "He gains weight so easily."

37. Correct answer - 2. The diagnosis is confirmed by sweat tests, which yield elevated chloride levels. Clients with CF seem to "taste salty." Option 1: Children who have CF generally have recurrent respiratory infections. Option 3: These childrens' stools are bulky and have a foul smell. They float in the toilet bowl because of the presence of undigested fat. Option 4: Children with CF generally suffer from failure to thrive.
CN: Physiological integrity

38. Which of the following measures should be a part of the care plan for a client in Bryant's traction?
    1. Encourage him to have high fiber intake.
    2. Keep his buttocks directly on the mattress.
    3. Release the weights that are part of his traction at regularly scheduled intervals.
    4. Provide him with foods low in fiber.

38. Correct answer - 1. A high fiber intake will prevent constipation caused by lack of mobility. Option 2: The buttocks should be raised so they do not rest on the mattress. Option 3: Once the weights have been attached, they should not be removed. Option 4: A high-fiber diet is provided to prevent constipation.
CN: Physiological integrity

39. A girl with anemia has a hemoglobin of 8 g/dl. Which measure is most important to include on the care plan?
    1. Teaching her active range-of-motion exercises.
    2. Planning rest periods between nursing activities.
    3. Checking her urine for presence of acetone.
    4. Restricting her intake of foods high in calcium.

39. Correct answer - 2. Because she is anemic, she will have little energy and needs periods of rest. Option 1: Exercise will only make her more fatigued and require her to expend more energy. Option 3: Anemia does not cause acetone to be present in the urine. Option 4: The child with anemia generally needs small, frequent feedings and needs no calcium restriction.
CN: Physiological integrity

40. If the developmental level is normal for a 5-week-old infant, which finding should the nurse expect while doing a physical assessment?
    1. Rooting reflex not present.
    2. Moro reflex not present.
    3. Rolls from abdomen to back.
    4. Turns head from side to side.

40. Correct answer - 4. This is appropriate behavior for a 5-week-old infant. Option 1: The rooting reflex is present until the infant is 4 months old. Option 2: The Moro reflex is present until the infant is 4 months old. Option 3: The infant is not expected to roll from abdomen to back until he is 5 months old.
CN: Health promotion and maintenance.

41. A child with CF has an order for oral pancreatic enzymes. At which time should they be administered?
    1. With meals
    2. Midway between meals
    3. At bedtime
    4. At least 2 hours before breakfast

41. Correct answer - 1. Enzymes are needed to assist in the absorption of nutrients. Option 2: The enzymes should reach the duodenum at the same time food does. Option 3: The enzymes are used to digest food and must be taken with food. Option 4: The enzymes must be taken with food.
    CN: Physiological integrity

42. A child with CF has chest physical therapy prescribed. The nurse knows that the therapy is successful if the client
    1. no longer coughs.
    2. does not take deep breaths.
    3. is able to breathe through his nose.
    4. is able to raise sputum.

42. Correct answer - 4. When chest physical therapy is done properly, chest secretions are moved up and out. Option 1: Exercises that stimulate coughing are encouraged. Option 2: Deep breaths aerate the lungs. Option 3: Congestion is in the chest, not the nose.
    CN: Physiological integrity

43. A 5-week-old boy is admitted to the hospital with a diagnosis of pyloric stenosis. The nurse should expect him to have which of the following symptoms?
    1. Bulging anterior fontanel.
    2. Projectile vomiting.
    3. Loose stools.
    4. Distended neck veins.

43. Correct answer - 2. The pylorus becomes partially blocked so that food does not empty properly into the duodenum. Peristalsis attempts to force the swallowed formula into the duodenum. When this effort proves ineffective, peristalsis reverses itself and projectile vomiting occurs. Option 1: A symptom of pyloric stenosis is dehydration and this causes a sunken fontanel. Option 3: Because dehydration is present, one would expect constipation, not loose stools. Option 4: Pyloric stenosis is a disease of the gastro-intestinal tract and does not cause this symptom.
    CN: Physiological integrity

44. You are admitting a 15-month-old boy who has bilateral otitis media and bacterial meningitis. Which is the *best* room for him?
    1. In isolation of a side hallway.
    2. In a private room near the nurse's station.
    3. In a room with another child who also has meningitis.
    4. In a room with two toddlers who have the croup.

44. Correct answer - 2. With meningitis, the child should be isolated for the first day and be close to where he can be observed frequently. Option 1 is too far away for frequent observation. Options 3 and 4 would present a hazard to the other clients.
    CN: Physiological integrity

45. A 10-year-old with CF has a respiratory infection. Albuterol, chest physiotherapy, and postural drainage are ordered. The rationale for this treatment is to
    1. decrease respiratory rate and mucus production.
    2. stimulate coughing and decrease oxygen saturation.
    3. dilate the bronchioles and clear secretions.
    4. increase the efficiency of the muscles of respiration and improve gas exchange.

45. Correct answer - 3. Albuterol therapy promotes bronchodilation, and chest physiotherapy clears the airway of excessive mucus. Option 1: Albuterol and chest physiotherapy do not decrease respiratory rate or the production of mucous. Option 2: Albuterol does not stimulate coughing. Chest physiotherapy does stimulate coughing, and decreasing oxygen saturation is contraindicated. Option 4: Albuterol relaxes the bronchial muscles, relieving bronchospasm and reducing airway resistance. It does *not* increase the efficiency of the muscles of respiration. Chest physiotherapy does improve respiratory muscle efficiency.
CN: Physiological integrity.

46. A 9-year-old child is admitted with a diagnosis of rheumatic fever. Which nursing intervention would *best* minimize arthralgia during the acute phase of illness?
    1. Immobilize his joints in functional positions using blanket rolls and pillows.
    2. Deep massage all extremities three times a day.
    3. Alternately apply hot and cold compresses and ambulate him.
    4. Provide full passive range of motion to all extremities four times a day.

46. Correct answer - 1. Immobilization in a functional position allows rest and healing. Option 2: Pain may be very intense and massage may only aggravate arthralgia. Option 3: Applying heat and cold and ambulating may aggravate arthralgia. During the acute phase the child needs bed rest. Option 4: This would not provide needed joint rest, be painful, and aggravate arthralgia.
CN: Physiological integrity

47. A 6-week-old girl is admitted to the pediatric unit following the surgical repair of a cleft lip. Which of the following should be included on her care plan?
    1. Postural drainage and early spoon feeding.
    2. Cleansing suture line and supine position or in infant seat.
    3. Mouth irrigations and prone position.
    4. Keep infant sedated and in elbow and ankle restraints.

47. Correct answer - 2. Cleansing suture line prevents inflammation or sloughing, which can interfere with optimal healing. Supine or infant seat are the best positions to prevent injury to the suture line. Option 1: Postural drainage is not necessary and may cause the baby to cry leading to stress on the suture line. Attempts at spoon feeding would injure suture line. Option 3: Mouth irrigations are not necessary and could injure the suture line. Prone position would injure suture line when the baby rubs her face against mattress. Option 4: Occasionally a very restless infant may need mild sedation but it is not usually warranted. Ankle restraints are not necessary and would cause undo stress for the baby. Elbow restraints can prevent the infant from putting hands and fingers in her mouth.
CN: Safe, effective care environment

48. A 7-year-old girl with sickle cell anemia is seen in the emergency department in vasoocclusive sickle-cell crisis. What is the *most* important nursing intervention?
    1. Administering antibiotics and obtaining a CBC.
    2. Getting a complete septic work-up and administering whole blood.
    3. Maintaining adequate hydration and oxygenation.
    4. Obtaining hemoglobin electrophoresis and providing pain relief.

48. Correct answer - 3. Maintaining adequate hydration is a primary nursing responsibility because dehydration enhances the sickling process, which in turn increases pain and gas exchange impairment. Option 1: These are not the first and immediate nursing actions; lab work and antibiotics, if indicated, can be done later. Option 2: A septic work-up to rule out an infection and the administration of blood, if necessary, do not take precedence over the immediate need for hydration and oxygenation. Option 4: Hemoglobin electrophoresis is a diagnostic test for detecting the homozygous and heterozygous forms of the disease--this child has already been diagnosed, so pain relief would follow the immediate goal of hydration and oxygenation.
CN: Physiological integrity

49. A 6-month-old baby with ventricular septal defect is seen in the pediatric ambulatory care center for a routine visit. The baby has been receiving oral digoxin since she was 1 month old. What information should the nurse get from the mother?
    1. Symptoms of headache, confusion and vertigo.
    2. The baby's daily record the respiratory rates.
    3. Any occurrence of anorexia and vomiting.
    4. Any development of macular exanthema and fever.

49. Correct answer - 3. The earliest signs of digoxin toxicity are anorexia, nausea (a 6-month-old might manifest these signs by refusing feeding), and vomiting. Option 1: Symptoms of headache, confusion and vertigo are difficult to identify in a 6-month-old and are of little value in assessing toxicity in infants. Option 2: Apical rates, not respiratory rates, should be obtained before digoxin administration. Option 4: Fever and macular exanthema are not associated with digoxin toxicity.
    CN: Physiological integrity

50. A child with leukemia is being treated with intrathecal methotrexate. Which of the following is a long-term adverse effect of this type of chemotherapy?
    1. Alopecia.
    2. Muscle atrophy.
    3. Hormonal dysfunction.
    4. Learning disabilities.

50. Correct answer - 4. Treatment that is directed toward the central nervous system, such as intrathecal chemotherapy (or cranial irradiation) has been shown to cause neurological and intellectual dysfunction in many childhood cancer survivors. Option 1 is a short term, uncommon adverse effect of methotrexate. Option 2 is not a short- or long-term adverse effect. Option 3 is a long-term adverse effect of radiation therapy.
    CN: Physiological integrity

51. A 2-day-old infant had a surgical repair of a myelomeningocele of the lumbosacral area. Which postoperative nursing intervention is *most* important in caring for this client?
    1. Assessing for impaired muscles of lower extremities.
    2. Accurately documenting I&O.
    3. Measuring and documenting head circumference.
    4. Assessing and observing for bradypnea and hypotension

51. Correct answer - 3. Hydrocephalus can occur as a complication of repair of a myelomeningocele and is manifested by an increase in head circumference, and/or tense, bulging fontanels. Option 1: The myelomeningocele, located in the lumbosacral region and the nerve supply to the lower extremities, was impaired before surgery. Option 2: Measuring I&O always is an important postoperative observation, but is not specific to this procedure. Option 4: Increased intracranial pressure can occur as a postoperative complication, causing blood pressure increase and fast, irregular respirations.
    CN: Physiological integrity

52. A 15-month-old child had surgery to correct Hirschsprung's disease (congenital aganglionic megacolon.) Which findings are most significant and should be reported *immediately?*
    1. Abdomen soft, stools brown and semi-formed, stoma decreasing in size.
    2. Temperature 98.1° F, abdomen soft, urine output 20 ml/hour.
    3. Abdomen flat, stoma red, presence of flatus.
    4. Temperature 96.4° F, abdomen distended, stoma red.

52. Correct answer - 4. Subnormal temperature, and distended abdomen may indicate the beginning of sepsis. Options 1, 2, and 3 all indicate expected or favorable observations.
CN: Physiological integrity

53. A child with tetralogy of Fallot is admitted for surgical correction. The results of preoperative blood work include: hemoglobin, 17 g/dl, and hematocrit, 58%. What is the correct interpretation of this data?
    1. The body is compensating for tissue hypoxia by increasing red blood cell production.
    2. The child is not anemic because the hemoglobin and hematocrit are elevated.
    3. These data are within normal limits.
    4. The child has hyperoxia because of the blood's increased oxygen carrying capacity.

53. Correct answer - 1. The body compensates for the tissue hypoxia, because of cyanotic heart disease, by stimulating the bone marrow to produce increased red blood cells. Option 2: Although an increased hemoglobin and hematocrit indicate that the child is not anemic, this statement does not accurately explain the reason for the increase. Option 3: The findings are elevated and not within normal limits. Option 4: A child with tetralogy of Fallot has hypoxemia because of decreased pulmonary blood flow.
CN: Physiological integrity

54. A 15-year-old girl is being treated in the clinic for iron- deficiency anemia. Because of her diagnosis, which of these questions would be *most* important for the nurse to ask?
    1. At what age did you start to menstruate?
    2. How many days do you menstruate each month?
    3. When did you last eat red meat?
    4. Do you include grains in your daily diet?

54. Correct answer - 2. Causes of iron-deficiency anemia may be malabsorption of iron, such as occurs in chronic diarrhea, malabsorption syndromes, and gastrectomy or blood loss by bleeding, (i.e., heavy menstruation or hemorrhage). Options 1, 3, and 4 have nothing to do with iron-deficiency anemia.
CN: Physiological integrity.

55. The mother of a 3-year-old boy reports that her child took "a lot of" Tylenol. She has a poison kit with syrup of ipecac and activated charcoal. Her home is approximately 1 hour's drive from the hospital. What should the nurse instruct the mother to do *first?*
    1. Administer 15 ml of syrup of ipecac orally, followed by 4 to 8 ounces of fluid to induce vomiting before bringing the child to the hospital.
    2. Administer 30 ml of syrup of ipecac orally, followed by 8 to 16 ounces of fluid to induce vomiting; don't leave for the hospital until he has vomited a large amount.
    3. Administer 10 g of activated charcoal, followed by 4 to 8 ounces of milk to absorb the toxin before bringing him to the hospital.
    4. Rush him to the hospital immediately, where professional treatment will be started as soon as he arrives.

55. Correct answer - 1. This is the correct dosage of ipecac and amount of fluid recommended to induce vomiting and eliminate the poison for a 3-year-old. Option 2: The amounts of ipecac and fluids are excessive for a preschooler. 90% of children vomit within 30 minutes of the appropriate dose of ipecac. Waiting for vomiting to occur would delay stomach gavage and administration of the antidote. Option 3: Activated charcoal should not be given in milk products and is used when evacuation of the stomach contents is unsafe. Option 4: Tylenol is rapidly absorbed from the GI tract, with peak levels 1 or 2 hours after ingestion. Failing to evacuate the stomach contents increase the risk of organ damage and death.
CN: Safe, effective care environment

56. A 1-month-old girl is admitted to the hospital with severe diarrhea. Which of these outcomes would be expected if her prescribed treatment is effective?
    1. Her fontanels are depressed.
    2. Her weight is stabilized.
    3. Her heart rate is about 115 bpm.
    4. Her urine specific gravity is decreased.

56. Correct answer - 3. Tachycardia occurs when a child is in acute dehydration caused by diarrhea. Also, oliguria and high urine specific gravity are common as dehydration progresses. Option 1:Infants who are dehydrated have a depressed fontanelle. Options 2: Weight would drop from fluid loss. Option 4: Urine specific gravity would be elevated because of high concentration.
CN: Physiological integrity.

57. A newborn girl weighed 6 pounds 2 ounces (2,778 grams) at birth. The nurse in the Well-Baby Clinic should expect the newborn to weigh which of these amounts at 12 months of age?
    1. 12 pounds (5,443 grams)
    2. 14 pounds (6,350 grams)
    3. 16 pounds (7,257 grams)
    4. 18 pounds (8,165 grams)

57. Correct answer - 4. Birth weight should triple by end of first year. Options 1, 2, and 3 are therefore incorrect.
CN: Health promotion and maintenance

58. Which of these findings would indicate that an infant in cardiac failure is having a toxic reaction to furosemide (Lasix)?
    1. Hyperactivity
    2. Increased salivation
    3. Tight hand grasp
    4. Lack of skin elasticity

58. Correct answer - 4. A client getting Lasix should be assessed for reduction of edema of feet, legs, and sacral area daily if medication is being used for heart failure. Excessive fluid loss will result in dehydration and poor skin turgor. Options 1 and 3: Central nervous system toxicity of Lasix results in fatigue, weakness, and paresthesia. Option 2: One of the adverse effects of Lasix is a dry mouth.
CN: Safe, effective environment

59. A 5-week-old infant was admitted for surgical repair of hypertrophic pyloric stenosis. Twenty-four hours following the pyloromyotomy, she began sterile water feedings, followed by clear liquids containing glucose and electrolytes. Now she is tolerating 30 to 45 ml of half-strength formula every 2 hours. She has not vomited, and her skin, incision, and color are good. Her TPR are normal. She begins to cry and thrashes her arms and legs. What is the *most* likely interpretation of this behavior?
    1. The baby is hungry.
    2. The baby is experiencing stranger anxiety.
    3. This is a normal postoperative response.
    4. The baby is experiencing incisional pain.

59. Correct answer - 4. An infant usually reacts to pain with loud crying and total body movement. It is likely that the infant is experiencing incisional pain. Option 1: There is no evidence that the infant has not been satisfied with the feedings, and the reaction described is more intense than a hunger response. Option 2: Stranger anxiety develops later in infancy. Option 3: The reaction described is too intense to be a normal response.
CN: Physiological integrity

60. A kindergarten teacher tells the school nurse that a 4-year-old boy in her class is preoccupied with looking at a little girl's genitalia. Which of these interpretations of the boy's behavior by the nurse is correct?
    1. He needs therapy because his behavior is abnormal.
    2. His behavior is within the normal parameters of children.
    3. He has evidently been exposed to such behavior in his home.
    4. His behavior is indicative of a sexually precocious child.

60. Correct answer - 2. According to Freud's theory, the phallic stage is from 3 to 6 years. During the phallic stage, the genitals become an interesting and sensitive area of the body. Children recognize differences between the sexes and become curious about the dissimilarities at this stage. Options 1, 3, and 4 are therefore incorrect.
CN: Health promotion and maintenance

61. The nurse should administer measles, mumps and rubella (MMR) vaccine by which of these routes?
    1. Subcutaneously
    2. Intramuscularly
    3. Intravenously
    4. Orally

61. Correct answer - 1. MMR is given subcutaneously. Options 2, 3, and 4 are incorrect on the basis of above statement.
CN: Physiological integrity

62. As a young boy who has a myelomeningocele reaches puberty, the nurse should discuss with the family which of these topics regarding a potential problem he might have?
    1. The development of his upper extremity muscles.
    2. The increase of protein in his diet.
    3. The risk of developing pathological fractures.
    4. The issue of his independence.

63. A 12-year-old boy with a history of sickle-cell anemia is admitted to the hospital in vaso-occlusive (thrombocytic) crisis. The boy, who is in bed, says to the nurse, "I'm really in pain. Do you think I should take something for it?" Which action should the nurse take?
    1. Encourage the boy to take medication when he has pain.
    2. Remind the boy that taking analgesics for pain can be addictive.
    3. Determine whether the boy understands that he must learn to tolerate the pain.
    4. Explain to the boy that if he ambulated, the pain would lessen.

64. A 5-year-old female child is admitted to the hospital with a diagnosis of meningitis. Which of these goals should have *priority* in the child's care plan? The child will
    1. experience no weight loss.
    2. be able to express her fears.
    3. remain seizure free.
    4. experience no cognitive loss.

65. A 1-year-old boy is admitted to the hospital with laryngotracheobronchitis (LTB). Which of these symptoms is likely to be present?
    1. Inspiratory stridor
    2. Extreme drowsiness
    3. A macular-papular rash on his chest
    4. A widening pulse pressure

62. Correct answer - 4. Adolescence is a particularly difficult time for children with myelomeningocele. The combination of altered body image, concerns about sexuality, and independence issues accentuate the typical adolescent turbulence. Options 1, 2, and 3: Issues that are emphasized earlier in the child's life to improve mobility, prevent fractures, and prevent obesity and are therefore incorrect.
CN: Health promotion and maintenance

63. Correct answer - 1. Pain is an expected finding during vaso-occlusive crisis and it is appropriate for children/adolescents experiencing pain to be given an analgesic. Options 2, 3, and 4 are therefore incorrect.
CN: Physiological integrity

64. Correct answer - 3. The child with a diagnosis of meningitis is overly sensitive to stimuli and needs to be in a quiet atmosphere. The temperature must be monitored. Seizures can occur because of meningeal irritation and cause further injury. Therefore, this goal must have priority. Options 1, 2 and 4 are therefore incorrect.
CN: Physiological integrity

65. Correct answer - 1. LTB is characterized by a sudden onset of inspiratory stridor, hoarseness, and a bark-like cough. These symptoms are caused by edema of the vocal cords and sub-glottal area. Option 2: The child is anxious and frightened, rather than drowsy. Options 3 and 4 are not symptoms of LTB.
CN: Physiological integrity

66. The mother of a 20-month-old child says to the
nurse in the clinic, "Since my son came home
from the hospital, he just clings to me." Which
of these ideas should the nurse include in her
response to the mother?
    1. "Allowing this behavior will just prolong
       the child's regression."
    2. "This is a normal reaction to the separation
       anxiety the child felt in the hospital."
    3. "This is normal behavior for a child of this
       age and would have occurred even if the
       child was not hospitalized."
    4. "It is important for you to find a male figure
       for the child to attach to at this time."

66. Correct answer - 2. Often after toddlers return
from a stay in the hospital--or even when the
mothers leave their toddlers for a while--the
toddlers react by regressing to more baby-like
behavior such as clinging to their mothers.
Mothers need to tolerate this behavior so that
the toddlers' trust can be reestablished. Options
1, 3, and 4 are therefore not correct.
CN: Health promotion and maintenance

67. A 10-year-old child is admitted to the hospital
with a diagnosis of acute lymphoblastic
leukemia. He is to be treated with a
combination of chemotherapeutic agents. One
of the nursing diagnoses that is appropriate for
the child is risk for injury related to decreased
platelet count. An appropriate outcome for that
diagnosis is
    1. improved appetite.
    2. increased white blood cell count.
    3. absence of bleeding.
    4. increased specific gravity of urine.

67. Correct answer - 3. When the platelet count is
lowered, the child is susceptible to bleeding.
This, in turn, places him at high risk for injury.
Therefore, a desired outcome is that no
bleeding will occur. Option 1: Although one
hopes that the child's appetite will improve,
that outcome is not directly related to the
diagnosis given. Options 2 and 4 also are not
directly related to the diagnosis.
CN: Physiological integrity

HOW TO SCORE AND USE THE DIAGNOSTIC PROFILE

In the top "QUESTION NUMBER" row of boxes, mark each question number you answered wrong. Under each question number, check the box in the "TEST TAKING SKILLS" section that is the most appropriate reason you answered the question incorrectly. Do the same for the "CLIENT NEED CATEGORIES" section. The client need category code follows the rationale. Total the number of check marks, by line, in the "Totals" column. This provides you with a profile of your weak areas that should be improve upon prior to taking the NCLEX-RN.

PERSONAL DIAGNOSTIC PROFILE

QUESTION NUMBER																					Totals

TEST-TAKING SKILLS

Misread the question																					
Missed important point																					
Forgot fact or concept																					
Applied wrong fact or concept																					
Drew wrong conclusion																					
Incorrectly evaluated distractors																					
Mistakenly selected answer choice																					
Read into question																					
Made a wrong guess																					
Misunderstood question																					

CLIENT NEED CATEGORIES

Safe, effective care environment																					
Physiological integrity																					
Psychosocial integrity																					
Health promotion and maintenance																					

CALCULATION OF SUBSCORES

After you score your test, determine your subscores in these client need categories by filling in the following grid.

CLIENT NEED

	Safe, effective care environment	Physiological integrity	Psychosocial integrity	Health promotion & maintenance
Number of questions	6	48	0	13
Number incorrect				
Number correct				
Percent correct*				

*To determine the percent correct in each category, divide the number of items answered correctly by the total number of items and multiply the result by 100.

Note: This is a short test with a limited sample of items in each category. Therefore, if a score in any category is less than 75% correct, further study is strongly advised.

CHAPTER 5

Medical/Surgical Nursing Skill Test

TAKING THIS SKILL TEST

Your Study Guide Module has instructed you to take the following skill test after you have completed your review of the clinical area. This test will give you needed experience in answering NCLEX-RN type questions and will give you a good idea of your competence in this clinical area.

The format of the skill test gives you instant feedback as you take it. Each question is in the left column. The correct answer with rationale is in the right column. As you read the question in the left-hand column, cover the right-hand column with an index card until you have selected your answer. Slide the card down, keeping remaining question answers covered. When you have completed the test, use the Personal Diagnostic Profile to record why you answered any question incorrectly.

If you scored lower than 75% on this skill test, you should analyze the reason and go back and do further review. You may also wish to consult a current nursing textbook for any areas that are unclear to you.

1. A client is scheduled for a magnetic resonance imaging (MRI) of an injured knee. What is the most accurate explanation of an MRI the nurse should give to the client?
   1. He will be given a dye to outline the knee tissues.
   2. He will have an examination using high-frequency sound waves.
   3. His injured knee will be placed in a doughnut-shaped magnet.
   4. He will hear no sounds during the examination.

2. A client who has just had a right total hip replacement complains of pain in the right calf. The pain is most likely related to which complication?
   1. Postoperative hemorrhage
   2. Pulmonary embolism
   3. Thrombophlebitis
   4. Wound infection

3. A hospitalized client has osteomyelitis caused by *Staphylococcus aureus*. What is the *best* intervention to prevent transmission of the organism to other clients?
   1. Using universal precautions during care.
   2. Keeping the client on bed rest with affected leg elevated.
   3. Administering ordered intravenous (I.V.) antibiotics.
   4. Providing hyperbaric oxygen treatments.

4. A client has been treated with busulfan (Myleran) for leukemia. His leucocyte count has declined to 10,000/mm^3 and the drug is stopped. His primary care nurse should tell him therapy will be restarted when his
   1. leucocyte count falls to 5,000/mm^3.
   2. lost hair grows back.
   3. hemoglobin falls to 8 g/dl.
   4. leucocyte count rises to 50,000/mm^3.

1. Correct answer - 3. Radio waves bombard the cells and the magnet helps realign the cells' ions to outline structures. Option 1 is incorrect as no dye is given. Option 2 describes ultrasound examination, not MRI. Option 4 is incorrect because there will be clicking sounds during the examination.
CN: Safe, effective care environment

2. Correct answer - 3. Thrombophlebitis is a common complication after total hip replacement. Options 1 and 4 also may occur but are not characteristic complaints of calf pain. Option 2 is secondary to thrombophlebitis and has different signs than calf pain.
CN: Physiological integrity

3. Correct answer - 1. Use of universal precautions is the only method to prevent nosocomial spread. All other options listed may also be used as treatments but don't prevent spread.
CN: Safe, effective care environment

4. Correct answer - 4. Chemotherapy should resume when the leucocyte count rises to 50,000/mm^3. Options 2 and 3 are not appropriate measures for resuming chemotherapy. Option 1 is a normal level. Waiting until then would allow the count to fall below normal risking the client for infection.
CN: Physiological integrity

5. A client with influenza A infection has rimantadine hydrochloride (Flumadine), 100 mg PO b.i.d. prescribed. The nurse explains that the client will need to take this drug for
   1. 3 days.
   2. 10 days.
   3. 7 days.
   4. 14 days.

6. A client who has had surgery to repair torn left knee ligaments calls the clinic to report that his left foot and toes feel numb and tingling. The nurse tells him to come to the emergency department immediately because his symptoms would indicate that he may have
   1. venous stasis.
   2. fat embolism.
   3. thrombophlebitis.
   4. compartment syndrome.

7. When planning care for a client who has had right hip replacement, the nurse should plan to have the client do toe-touch weight-bearing on the right leg on which postoperative day?
   1. The first day
   2. The second day
   3. The fifth day
   4. The tenth day

8. Who should be permitted to visit a client who is getting external radiation therapy to her thoracic and lumbar spine because of metastatic breast cancer?
   1. Her granddaughter, who is 3 months pregnant.
   2. Her husband, who is recovering from the flu.
   3. Her grandson, his wife, and four children.
   4. Her sister, who has frequent respiratory infections

5. Correct answer - 3. When used to treat influenza A, rimantadine should be taken for 7 days after symptoms appear. Option 1: Taking the drug for a shorter time may not destroy all the viruses. Options 2 and 4: Taking the drug for more time has not been clinically justified.
CN: Physiological integrity

6. Correct answer - 4. Numbness and tingling are two signs of compartment syndrome. Option 1: Swelling and "heaviness" are signs of venous stasis. Option 2: Symptoms would likely be hypoxia, tachypnea, and tachycardia from fat embolus lodging in lungs. Option 3: This is characterized by pain, swelling, and warmth.
CN: Physiological integrity

7. Correct answer - 2. Toe-touch weight-bearing should wait until vital signs are stabilized and there is sufficient wound healing. With "stepped up" recovery time, health care providers often order weight-bearing on day 2. Option 1: This is too soon. Option 3: Current quick recovery times make the fifth day too late for weight-bearing. Option 4: Toe-touch weight-bearing begins on the second postoperative day. The client is discharged on day 7.
CN: Physiological integrity

8. Correct answer - 1. External radiation poses to danger to the granddaughter, and she would pose no health threat to the client. Option 2: The husband should not visit until he is fully recovered from the flu because of risk of infection. Option 3: Large crowds and children who could possibly spread URIs should be avoided. Option 4: The sister could spread respiratory infections.
CN: Safe, effective care environment

9. Ibuprofen (Advil), a non-steroidal antiinflammatory drug (NSAID), should not be given to clients who have a history of
   1. hypotension.
   2. rheumatoid arthritis.
   3. fever.
   4. gastric ulcers.

9. Correct answer - 4. Non-steroidal antiinflammatory drugs can cause gastrointestinal (GI) upset and may worsen ulcer disease. Option 1: This class of drugs can cause slight fluid-related hypertension. Option 2: This class of drug is indicated for the antiinflammatory action. Option 3: This class of drugs has antipyretic properties.
   CN: Physiological integrity

10. A 52-year-old man has been on chemotherapy for metastatic cancer. His platelets are $20,000/mm^3$, hemoglobin is 10 g/dl, and hematocrit is 42%. He is admitted for dehydration and is to get I.V. fluids. Which nursing intervention would be *most* appropriate?
    1. Start the I.V. with a 16-gauge catheter.
    2. Apply pressure on an unsuccessful venipuncture site for 2 or 3 minutes.
    3. Give all analgesics by the intramuscular (I.M.) route.
    4. Wrap the infusion site and the area around it with gauze.

10. Correct answer - 4. He is prone to bleeding, and safety precautions should be taken to protect the integrity of the skin and prevent bleeding from puncture site. Option 1 is a large-bore catheter; the smallest catheter should be used to prevent bleeding. Option 2: Pressure should be applied for 10 minutes or until the bleeding stops when dealing with a client with such a low platelet count. Option 3: The I.M. route should be avoided, if possible, because of bleeding potential. The oral route or I.V. route is desirable.
    CN: Safe, effective care environment

11. A 46-year-old man is being treated for hepatitis B. He is jaundiced and is complaining of weakness. What should be included in his care plan?
    1. Rest periods following small, frequent meals.
    2. A low-protein diet.
    3. Let the client select his own foods.
    4. Provide for regular exercise.

11. Correct answer - 1. Rest periods are needed to help the client deal with weakness and fatigue. Small, frequent meals are needed because he may be anorexic. Large meals usually further decrease appetite. Option 2: A diet high in protein is recommended to enhance recovery of injured liver cells. Option 3: The client needs a high-protein diet. Choices can be made from a high-protein diet menu. Option 4: Rest, not exercise, is indicated during the acute phase of the disease.
    CN: Physiological integrity

12. What is the primary purpose of applying ice to a knee injured in a football game?
    1. Decreases bleeding.
    2. Brings about vasodilation.
    3. Increases venous return.
    4. Decreases recovery time.

13. A client on hemodialysis has had surgery to form an arteriovenous fistula. What is most important for the nurse to be aware of when providing care for the client?
    1. Do not use a stethoscope for auscultating the fistula.
    2. Encourage him to exercise after the dialysis treatment.
    3. Do not take blood pressures on the affected arm.
    4. Tell him that there will be no pain starting dialysis.

14. Crutchfield tongs have just been inserted for a client who has had a cervical neck injury. When evaluating the care plan, which of these measures should have been included on a daily basis?
    1. Cleansing and applying antibiotic ointment to the pin sites to prevent infection.
    2. Turning the screw a ¼-inch to relieve pressure at the pin sites.
    3. Removing the weights to assess neck mobility and sensation periodically.
    4. Keeping the neck in a position of flexion to promote stabilization of the spine.

12. Correct answer - 1. Applications of ice (cryotherapy) or cold packs causes vasoconstriction, thereby decreasing bleeding. Option 2: Vasoconstriction occurs, not vasodilation. Option 3 is accomplished by elevating the affected leg. Option 4: There are many factors that affect recovery time.
CN: Physiological integrity

13. Correct answer - 3. Pressure on the fistula or on the extremity can decrease blood flow and precipitate clotting. Option 1: Auscultating a bruit in the fistula is one way to determine patency. Option 2: Typically, clients feel very fatigued immediately after hemodialysis because of the rapid change in fluid and electrolyte status. Option 4: Although the area over the fistula may have diminished sensation, the needle stick is still painful.
CN: Safe, effective care environment

14. Correct answer - 1. With Crutchfield tongs, holes are made in the client's skull. Therefore, infection at the tong sites is a potential problem and prevention measures must be instituted. Options 2, 3 and 4: Turning the screw of the device and removing the weights are contraindicated at this time. The screw should never be adjusted, and the traction should be maintained at all times. After reduction of the cervical spine has occurred, however, the weights may *gradually* be removed. The client's neck should *never* be flexed; it should be maintained in a neutral or extension position.
CN: Safe, effective care environment

15. A client had a total hip replacement on the previous day. Prior to morning care, the nurse makes all of the following observations of the client. Which one requires *immediate* intervention?
    1. Her wound drainage system (Hemovac) contains about 20 ml of dark red drainage.
    2. She has anti-emboli hose on both of her lower extremities.
    3. Her hip is in an adducted position.
    4. The head of her bed is elevated 30 degrees.

15. Correct answer - 3. Following a total hip replacement, the position of the hip should be in abduction to prevent dislocating the hip prosthesis. Options 1, 2, and 4: Drainage of 200 to 500 ml of bloody fluid should be expected in the first 24 hours postoperatively, plus the drainage is dark red, which indicates that it is not fresh bleeding. To prevent thromboembolism, anti-emboli hose are ordered for both extremities; and the client's head can be elevated up to 45 degrees. A higher head elevation would acutely flex the hip, which could dislocate the hip prosthesis.
CN: Safe, effective care environment

16. A client is scheduled to have an I.V. pyelogram (IVP) because it is suspected that he has renal calculi. Prior to the test, which of these measures should be included in his care?
    1. Collecting his urine for 24 hours.
    2. Checking him for allergies.
    3. Encouraging him to eat foods high in calcium 2 days before the procedure.
    4. Informing him that he may have a metallic taste during the procedure.

16. Correct answer - 2. Because a dye is injected prior to the test, determining the client's history of allergies--especially to iodine or shellfish--is essential. Options 1: A 24-hour urine collection is not necessary for a IVP. Option 3: A high-calcium diet is required for an IVP. Option 4: There is no metallic taste during an IVP.
CN: Safe, effective care environment

17. A client who is being prepared for a gastrectomy is ordered atropine sulfate preoperatively. The chief purpose of the medication for him is to
    1. depress muscular activity at the duodenum.
    2. reduce the amount of general anesthesia required.
    3. prevent reflex tachycardia during general anesthesia.
    4. decrease respiratory secretions.

17. Correct answer - 4. When anticholinergic medications like atropine sulfate are prescribed preoperatively, they are expected to reduce respiratory secretions. Options 1: Although atropine sulfate relaxes the upper GI tract, it is not the chief reason why it is given. Option 2: Other medications, like opiates, are given for this purpose. Option 3: Another purpose of atropine sulfate is to prevent reflex bradycardia during general anesthesia.
CN: Physiological integrity

18. A client has just been told that she has hypothyroidism. Because of her diagnosis, which of these goals would likely be developed for her care plan?
    1. To decrease sensory stimulation.
    2. To maintain normal body temperature.
    3. To regain normal urinary elimination patterns.
    4. To prevent pathological fractures.

18. Correct answer - 2. Clients with hypothyroidism frequently have subnormal temperatures and are especially sensitive to cold and drafts, often complaining of cold even in a warm temperature. Options 1, 3, and 4: These clients may have dull mental processes and subdued emotional responses. If anything, sensory stimulation may need to be increased. Hypothyroidism does not directly affect the urinary tract system, nor does it encourage pathological fractures.
    CN: Physiological integrity.

19. A client has gone to the operating room for a subtotal thyroidectomy. In preparing her room for her return from surgery, it would be essential to have which of the following equipment at her bedside?
    1. Overhead trapeze.
    2. Tracheostomy tray.
    3. Surgical (Kelly) clamps.
    4. Humidifier.

19. Correct answer - 2. Occasionally, difficulty in respirations occurs as a result of edema of the glottis or an injury to the recurrent laryngeal nerve. Thus, a tracheostomy set should be at the bedside. Options 1, 3, and 4: None of this equipment needs to be available.
    CN: Safe, effective care environment

20. A client has had a subtotal thyroidectomy. Which of these findings, if it occurred, would clearly indicate that he has an injury to his recurrent laryngeal nerve?
    1. Throat pain
    2. Difficulty swallowing
    3. Presence of Chvostek's sign
    4. Inability to speak

20. Correct answer - 4. Voice changes, i.e., hoarseness, in addition to respiratory difficulties, indicate such damage. Options 1 and 2: The glossopharyngeal nerve (cranial nerve 9) is largely responsible for swallowing, gag, and cough reflexes as well as some throat pain. Option 4: Chvostek's sign is an indication of hypercalcemia, which may occur after a thyroidectomy. It is due to the removal of the parathyroid gland.
    CN: Physiological integrity

21. A client is admitted to the hospital with symptoms suggestive of acute pancreatitis. To help establish a definitive diagnosis, additional information definitely should be collected to determine if the client has an elevated level of serum
    1. acid phosphatase.
    2. creatine phosphokinase.
    3. amylase.
    4. sodium.

21. Correct answer - 3. The primary diagnostic tests for acute pancreatitis are serum amylase and lipase, and urinary amylase levels. The serum amylase level is the criterion most commonly used. It usually is elevated early and remains elevated for a few days. Options 1, 2, and 4: Elevation of these levels are associated with other conditions. For example, cancer of the prostate (acid phosphatase), musculoskeletal injury or disease (creatine phosphokinase), and impaired renal function and dehydration (sodium). Note that although the sodium may be elevated in acute pancreatitis because the client may be dehydrated from vomiting, it does not establish a definitive diagnosis as stated in the question.
CN: Physiological integrity

22. A client is to get supplemental nutrition by means of a nasogastric tube. The order is for the client to receive 200 ml of blenderized foods every 4 hours. Prior to instilling the feeding into the client, a correct step would include ensuring that
    1. appropriate sterile equipment is available.
    2. the feeding is warmed to body temperature.
    3. the client's head is elevated at least 30 degrees.
    4. residual stomach contents are aspirated and discarded.

22. Correct answer - 3. To prevent aspiration, the client's head should be elevated. Options 1, 2, and 4: Sterile equipment is not needed for nasogastric tube feedings; the feedings should be warmed to *room* temperature and not body temperature; and residual contents in the stomach should be reinstalled to prevent electrolyte imbalance.
CN: Physiological integrity

23. Indomethacin (Indocin) is prescribed for a client who has rheumatoid arthritis. The client should be observed for adverse effects of the medication, which include
    1. dizziness.
    2. hirsutism.
    3. hiccups.
    4. dry skin.

23. Correct answer - 1. Indocin has many adverse effects, including dizziness. Options 2, 3, and 4 are not adverse effects of this drug.
CN: Physiological integrity

24. A client who has chronic renal failure is getting hemodialysis treatments. The treatment has been effective if which of these results is obtained?
    1. The client's serum electrolytes are close to normal.
    2. The client's glomerular filtration rate is increased.
    3. The client's urine has fewer red blood cells.
    4. The client's kidneys have less physiological change.

24. Correct answer - 1. The major purposes of dialysis are to remove fluid, toxic substances, and body wastes, normally secreted by healthy kidneys. As renal function declines, the end products of protein metabolism accumulate in the blood. The client tends to retain sodium and water. Other imbalances occur in serum calcium and phosphate levels. Thus, the treatment is effective if serum electrolyte values approach normal. Options 2, 3, and 4: Hemodialysis itself neither improves kidney functioning nor alters the natural course of the underlying kidney disease.
    CN: Physiological integrity

25. A client who has recently been diagnosed as having type 1 (insulin-dependent) diabetes mellitus (DM), is being taught about the food exchange lists prepared by the American Dietetic Association (ADA). The instruction has been effective if he selects which of these foods as an appropriate exchange for white rice?
    1. Egg
    2. Tomato
    3. Apple
    4. Bread

25. Correct answer - 4. In the ADA lists, foods are divided into six basic groups (some with subgroups): Milk, vegetables, fruit, starch/bread, meat, and fat. Each food item within a group or subgroup contains about the same food value as any other food item in that group, allowing for exchange within groups, thus providing for variety in food choices as well as food value control. Both rice and bread are in the starch/bread group. Options 1, 2, and 3: Eggs are in the meat group, tomatoes in the vegetable group, and apples in the fruit group.
    CN: Physiological integrity

26. A client has a total colectomy and ileostomy. He has a disposable ileostomy drainage bag in place. The nurse should ensure that the appliance fits closely around the stoma to prevent
    1. wound dehiscence.
    2. abdominal fistulas.
    3. incisional herniation.
    4. peristomal skin irritation.

26. Correct answer - 4. The most common complication following this surgery is peristomal skin irritation, which is caused by drainage leaking through the stoma. Options 1, 2, and 3: A properly fitting appliance would not prevent these problems.
    CN: Physiological integrity

27. As part of a nursing audit, a nurse is evaluating the care plan of a client who has been admitted in Addisonian crisis. Which one of these measures should have been included in the client's care on admission?
    1. Testing each of his voidings for protein.
    2. Maintaining the temperature of his room at 60° F.
    3. Placing him on reverse isolation.
    4. Assessing him for the presence of edema.

27. Correct answer - 3. Clients in Addisonian crisis should be protected from infection. Placing the client on reverse isolation helps to achieve this goal. Options 1, 2, and 4: There is no need to check urine for protein. Clients do need to be protected from stress which includes environmental temperature extremes. In this case, the room would be too cold. Finally, clients in Addisonian crisis typically have fluid volume deficit and thus would not need to be assessed for edema.
CN: Safe, effective care environment

28. A client goes to his health care provider because of symptoms suggestive of rheumatoid arthritis. To help confirm the diagnosis, the nurse should expect the client to have which of these blood test results?
    1. Elevated erythrocyte sedimentation rate (ESR)
    2. Negative C-reactive protein
    3. Increased red blood cell (RBC) count
    4. Decreased myoglobin

28. Correct answer - 1. In rheumatoid arthritis, the ESR is significantly elevated because of the presence of inflammation. Options 2, 3, and 4: For the client with rheumatoid arthritis, the C-reactive protein is positive and the RBC count decreased. Myoglobin results are not pertinent for rheumatoid arthritis.
CN: Physiological integrity

29. Which statement best indicates a client with hepatitis B understands the discharge teaching?
    1. "My family knows if I became tired and start vomiting, I may be getting sick again."
    2. "I now can never get hepatitis again."
    3. "I'll never have a liver problem again, even if I drink alcohol."
    4. "I can safely give blood 3 months after I'm discharged."

29. Correct answer - 1. Clients can have relapses of hepatitis B with symptoms of fatigue, nausea and vomiting, and bleeding or bruising. Option 2: Symptoms of hepatitis B can recur. Option 3: Alcohol is metabolized by the liver and should be avoided by a client with hepatitis B. Option 4: Clients with hepatitis should be instructed not to donate blood.
CN: Health promotion and maintenance

30. A 20-year-old man is prescribed cefpodoxime proxetil (Vantin) for a urinary infection. What teaching is *most* important to give him?
    1. Limit fluid intake while on this medication.
    2. Take medication on an empty stomach.
    3. Take medication with food.
    4. Take an antacid if nausea occurs.

31. A client is being treated for hepatitis A. In teaching assistive personnel and the family how to protect themselves from being infected, which instruction should the nurse stress?
    1. Avoid contact with the client's blood, body fluids, and needles.
    2. Keep immunization status current by receiving hepatitis vaccine.
    3. Avoid contact with anyone who has a cold.
    4. Wear a mask when providing care for the client.

32. A nurses' aide approaches the nurse and says, "I want to know who has AIDS on this unit. I don't go in those rooms. That is catching." Which action, by the nurse, would be *most* appropriate?
    1. Identify clients with acquired immunodeficiency syndrome (AIDS) and assign an RN to give care.
    2. Identify the AIDS clients and accompany the aide to their rooms.
    3. Explain that casual contact doesn't cause AIDS, and monitor the aide's activities.
    4. Give the aide latex gloves, explain universal precautions, and monitor care activities.

30. Correct answer - 3. Taking with food increases absorption of drug and minimizes adverse GI reactions. Option 1: Fluid intake should be *increased* to ensure adequate hydration. Option 2 is exactly opposite of the correct answer. Option 4: Antacids interact with Vantin, decreasing its absorption.
CN: Safe, effective care environment

31. Correct answer - 2. Hepatitis vaccine is available for hepatitis A. Caregivers who have close contacts with clients with hepatitis A should be vaccinated for hepatitis A. Option 1: Although hepatitis B, C, and D are spread by contaminated needles and other equipment that comes in contact with infected body fluids, the hepatitis A is primarily transmitted person-to-person through fecal contamination. For all clients, universal precautions should be taken in handling body fluids, and needles. Option 3: Being in contact with someone who has URI or even acquiring a respiratory infection would not put a caregiver at risk. Hepatitis A is not airborne. Option 4: Hepatitis A is not transmitted via the respiratory system.
CN: Safe, effective care environment

32. Correct answer - 3. Casual contact has not been identified as a mode of transmission, and making sure that all clients get appropriate care is a nursing responsibility. Options 1 and 2 violate client confidentiality. Option 4: Universal precautions, the use of latex gloves, is indicated only when the risk of contact with blood or body fluids exists. This risk would not exist for someone giving casual care.
CN: Safe, effective care environment

33. A female client has been returned to the unit after biliary tract surgery. She has a T-tube in place. What should the nurse do with the T-tube?
    1. Clamp the tube.
    2. Irrigate the tube with normal saline, as needed.
    3. Place the tube to gravity drainage.
    4. Connect the tube to intermittent suction.

34. A client who has just returned from surgery to repair a leg fracture asks the nurse what can be done to decrease the pain in his leg. What is the nurse's *best* response?
    1. "If you lie quietly, it should decrease quickly."
    2. "Hold your ice bags over the painful area."
    3. "I'll give you some pain medication to relieve it."
    4. "I need to further assess your leg before deciding."

35. A client with myasthenia gravis has been taking neostigmine sulfate (Prostigmin) and digoxin. She develops a leg abscess and the health care provider prescribes clindamycin phosphate (Cleocin). The nurse reviews the client's medication history and questions the drug order because she knows clindamycin enhances the action of
    1. beta-adrenergic blocking drugs.
    2. antiarrhythmic drugs.
    3. anticonvulsant drugs.
    4. neuromuscular blocking drug.

36. Which assessment finding would be an early sign of shock?
    1. Increased restlessness
    2. Increased pulse rate
    3. Decreased blood pressure
    4. Decreased urine output

---

33. Correct answer - 3. The T-tube is inserted to let bile drain from the traumatized common bile duct. A gravity drainage system is used. Options 1, 2, and 4: Connecting the tube to suction, clamping or irrigating the T-tube could harm the surgical site.
CN: Safe, effective care environment

34. Correct answer - 4. Having only one piece of data is insufficient to serve as a base for more definitive action. You need to gather more data to provide the safest client care. Completing a neurovascular assessment should give you more information on which to base your response. Options 1, 2, and 3 all lack data.
CN: Safe, effective care environment

35. Correct answer - 4. Clindamycin enhances the action of neuromuscular blocking agents by blocking neuromuscular transmission. Options 1, 2, and 3: There is no known interaction with antiarrhythmics, anticonvulsants, or beta-adrenergic blocking drugs.
CN: Safe, effective care environment

36. Correct answer - 1. Restlessness is a sign of cerebral irritability caused by decreased cerebral circulation with resultant cerebral hypoxia. Options 2, 3 and 4 all are later signs of shock.
CN: Physiological integrity

37. A client had surgical repair of a femoral fracture and asks how he can help in his recovery. What is your *best* response?
    1. "Relax your muscles so you won't fight the traction."
    2. "Take deep breaths to increase the oxygen to your legs."
    3. "Repeat the quad setting exercises every 2 hours."
    4. "Choose high-protein and high-carbohydrate foods from your menu."

37. Correct answer - 3. Performing "quad setting" exercises increases the blood flow through the injured area, which helps resolve the inflammation while helping maintain the muscle strength and mass needed for crutch walking later. Option 1: Spasms are likely to be present because of injury, so muscle relaxation may not be possible. Option 2: Deep breathing helps peripheral circulation, but is not the best option available. Option 4: Improving nutritional status is specific to bone healing, but it is not the best of the options available.
CN: Physiological integrity

38. A 78-year-old female has cardiac failure. As a home health nurse, you are visiting her to evaluate her compliance with medication therapy. Which of the following factors *best* indicates she is complying with digitalis therapy?
    1. Her ability to correctly count her radial pulse.
    2. Her weight gain of 2 pounds in less than a week.
    3. An apical heart rate of 100 or greater.
    4. Absence of a pericardial friction rub.

38. Correct answer - 1. Recurrence of cardiac failure is preventable if clients are taught to comply with drug therapy. Correctly checking her pulse daily prevents the chance of digitalis toxicity. Option 2: Weight gain of 2 pounds in a short period could be a sign of fluid overload or indicate digitalis has not been taken. Option 3: Apical rate greater than 100 could indicate digitalis has not been taken. Option 4: Pericardial friction rub occurs in pericarditis and has no relationship to digitalis therapy.
CN: Physiological integrity

39. A 65-year-old man has just been admitted with a myocardial infarction (MI). He is getting nasal oxygen at 2 liters, an I.V. at keep-vein-open rate, and morphine sulfate 2 mg I.V. prn for chest pain. He is on continuous cardiac monitoring and is very apprehensive. Which intervention would *best* reduce his apprehension?
    1. Explain the medical equipment being used and his nursing care.
    2. Pull the curtain around the bed and reduce unit noise.
    3. Give him literature that explains hospital policies.
    4. Explain the call light and put it within his reach.

39. Correct answer - 1. Apprehension may be best relieved by remaining with the client and explaining the type of care he will receive. Option 2: Isolation is likely to increase his anxiety. Option 3: Highly anxious people have difficulty focusing on written materials. Option 4: This action should *follow* an explanation of equipment and nursing care.
CN: Psychosocial integrity

40. A client who is getting oral anticoagulants has overheard her health care provider say that her prothrombin time (protime) is 23 seconds. She asks the nurse if this is good. What is the nurse's *best* response?
    1. "Your prothrombin time is just right for a client being anticoagulated."
    2. "Your prothrombin time is prolonged; your medicine dose will be decreased."
    3. "Your prothrombin time is too low; you will need more anticoagulation."
    4. "Your health care provider will answer that question."

40. Correct answer - 1. The normal prothrombin time is 11 or 12 seconds. For effective anticoagulation, the protime should be 1½ to 2½ times normal. Options 2 and 3: Pro time is within the therapeutic range for a client being anticoagulated. Option 4: The client has a right to information and it is within the nurse's role to provide it.
CN: Physiological integrity

41. The nurse is teaching a client with osteoporosis to minimize eating foods low in calcium and high in phosphorus. Which foods should he avoid?
    1. Cheese and skim milk
    2. Red meats and processed foods
    3. Dark green vegetables
    4. Salmon and broccoli

41. Correct answer - 2. These foods are low in calcium and high in phosphorus. A calcium/phosphorus ratio of 1:1 is considered therapeutic. Options 1, 3, and 4: These foods are high in calcium and should be encouraged.
CN: Physiological integrity

42. When assessing a client with chronic airflow limitation, which of the following would the nurse expect to find?
    1. Dyspnea, cough, bradycardia
    2. Wheezing, tachycardia, restlessness
    3. Barrel chest, tachycardia, hypertension
    4. Hypotension, confusion, weight gain

42. Correct answer - 2. Wheezing results from air being expired against a collapsed airway. Tachycardia results from hypoxia. Restlessness results from cerebral hypoxia. Option 1: Chronic airflow limitation results in tachycardia from hypoxia. Option 3: Hypertension is not present in chronic airflow limitation unless the client has other underlying problems. Option 4: Clients with this disorder often experience anorexia with subsequent weight loss, not weight gain.
CN: Physiological integrity

43. A client with advanced human immunodeficiency virus (HIV) has not responded to zidovudine. Stavudine (Zerit), an antiviral drug, has been prescribed. The nurse teaches the client that he should take only the number of capsules prescribed because the dose is specific for his
    1. weight.
    2. age.
    3. sex.
    4. physical condition.

43. Correct answer - 1. The adult dosage for stavudine is based on weight: 40 mg PO q12h for those weighing 60 kg or more; 30 mg PO q12h for those weighing less. Options 2, 3, and 4 are not factors used in determining dosage.
CN: Safe, effective care environment

44. A client who has had a segmental left lung resection is returned from surgery with a left posterior-lateral chest tube attached to a closed chest drainage system. Which of the following would indicate that the drainage system is working properly?
    1. The water-seal chamber is bubbling steadily and constantly.
    2. The client shows signs of a beginning pneumothorax.
    3. Water in the water-seal chamber moves up with inspiration and down with expiration.
    4. There is no fluctuation in the water-seal chamber when the client coughs.

45. A client is 3 days postoperative after a segmental lung resection. A chest x-ray confirms the lung has re-expanded. The surgeon is preparing to remove the chest tube. Which of the following instructions should the nurse give the client during the removal of the chest tube?
    1. Inhale deeply and exhale frequently.
    2. Do Valsalva maneuver.
    3. Intermittently cough.
    4. Breath normally.

46. A client taking a daily anticoagulant wants to take an NSAID for frequent headaches. He asks the nurse if the NSAID will have any effect on his anticoagulant. Which response is *best?*
    1. "No, the two drugs won't affect each other."
    2. "You may have GI upset, but your protime will not be effected."
    3. "The amount of anticoagulant may need to be decreased to account for an increase in your protime."
    4. "The ibuprofen will antagonized the anticoagulant so your protime will decrease."

44. Correct answer - 3. The fluid fluctuates upward upon inspiration and downward with exhalation, indicating effective communication between the pleural cavity and the drainage chamber; therefore, patency is present. Option 1 indicates the presence of a pleural air leak. Option 2: Signs and symptoms of tension pneumothorax indicate air is trapped in the pleural space. Option 4: With a patent chest tube, water in the water-seal chamber would fluctuate when the client coughs.
CN: Physiological integrity

45. Correct answer - 2. Preventing air from entering the pleural cavity as the tube is withdrawn is important. The Valsalva maneuver accomplishes this. Options 1 and 4 let air enter the pleural cavity during the removal of the chest tube. Option 3: Coughing causes jarring and interferes with the removal of the chest tube.
CN: Physiological integrity

46. Correct answer - 3. NSAIDs may increase the actions of anticoagulants and increase the protime. Options 1, 2, and 4 are not correct.
CN: Physiological integrity

47. A female client with heart failure was placed on daily digoxin 0.25 mg PO and Lasix 40 mg PO qd. During a home visit, she tells the nurse she feels weak and often feels her heart "flutter." What is the nurse's *best* response?
    1. Tell her to be less active and to rest more often.
    2. Tell her to stop taking her digoxin.
    3. Tell her you will report the symptoms and request a potassium level be done.
    4. Tell her to avoid foods and drinks that have caffeine in them.

47. Correct answer - 3. Lasix is a potassium-wasting diuretic. A low potassium level may cause weakness and palpitations. Option 1 will not help if she is hypokalemic, which can cause life-threatening arrhythmias. Option 2: There is no basis for such instructions. Option 4: She probably should avoid caffeine but that does not address her symptoms of potassium depletion. CN: Physiological integrity

48. While walking in the hall with the nurse, a client with epilepsy has an aura and begins to fall to the floor with a generalized motor seizure. What should the nurse do *first?*
    1. Administer an ordered anticonvulsant immediately.
    2. Elevate his head.
    3. Help him into the supine position.
    4. Hyperextend his head.

48. Correct answer - 3. To protect the client from injury while falling, the nurse should help him immediately to a supine position. Option 1: The client is probably taking routine medication for epilepsy. Even if he requires medication, it would not be the first thing the nurse would do during a seizure. Option 2: No attempt should be made to position the head; just protect the client from injury. Option 4: The head should not be hyperextended because of the danger of aspiration or choking on secretions. CN: Physiological integrity

49. A client with AIDS has developed *Pneumocystis carinii* pneumonia. On admission to the hospital, his health care provider orders pentamidine isethionate (Pentam 300), 4 mg/kg I.V. daily for 14 days. What is the most important intervention the nurse should include in the client's care plan?
    1. Administer over a 1-hour period, keeping client in a semi-Fowler's position.
    2. Administer over 30 minutes, keeping the client supine.
    3. Administer by bolus, keeping client supine.
    4. Administer over a 1-hour period, keeping client supine.

49. Correct answer - 4. Pentamidine should be infused over a 1-hour period with the client supine to minimize hypotension and arrhythmias. Option 1, 2, and 3: These interventions could cause severe hypotension. CN: Health promotion and maintenance

50. A 19-year-old man has a history of seizures and is having his annual evaluation. The client takes phenytoin sodium (Dilantin) 100 mg t.i.d. to control his seizures. While doing a physical assessment, the nurse should pay special attention to
    1. his musculoskeletal development.
    2. his gastrointestinal function.
    3. the condition of his gums.
    4. his psychosocial development.

50. Correct answer - 3. Dilantin causes hypertrophy of the gums. Options 1, 2, and 4: There is no particular risk of impairment of any of these systems in clients with seizure disorders who are taking Dilantin.
    CN: Physiological integrity

51. Twenty-four hours after suffering a cerebral vascular accident (CVA) a client has right side hemiplegia. Which neurologic deficits are closely associated with this type of hemiplegia?
    1. Trouble speaking and understanding
    2. Loss of consciousness
    3. Inability to see to the left
    4. Poor judgment, impulsive behavior

51. Correct answer - 1. Expressive and receptive dysphasias are associated with damage to the left hemisphere, where the dominant speech centers are in most people. Because motor tracks cross in the medulla, a right-sided hemiplegia indicates a left-sided brain injury. Option 2: Loss of consciousness can result from any type of CVA. Option 3: A client with a left-sided CVA may have difficulty with right-sided vision. Option 4: Poor judgment and impulsive behavior are associated with damage to the right hemisphere.
    CN: Physiological integrity

52. Which nursing intervention is *best* for a client hospitalized with severe cirrhosis?
    1. Keeping the bed flat to lessen pressure of abdominal ascites.
    2. Keeping the client on medical isolation to prevent infection.
    3. Assisting him with pre-meal mouth care to stimulate eating.
    4. Observing him for hyperkalemia related to diuretic use.

52. Correct answer - 3. Clients with cirrhosis usually have an unpleasant mouth odor because of ammonia excretion. Option 1: The bed should be in semi-Fowler's position to aid respiratory functions. Option 2 is not appropriate for clients with cirrhosis. Option 4: Hypokalemia is common with diuretic use, not hyperkalemia.
    CN: Physiological integrity

53. Which finding would be within normal limits (WNL) when assessing a client with a traumatic leg injury?
    1. His foot is edematous.
    2. His foot is discolored.
    3. He identifies which toe is being felt.
    4. His capillary refill of 4 to 6 seconds.

53. Correct answer - 3. Normally a person should be able to sense separate digits when felt. Options 1 and 2 may be *expected* findings after a traumatic injury, but are not WNL. Option 4: Normal capillary refill is 2 to 4 seconds.
    CN: Safe, effective care environment

54. A 65-year-old female with osteoarthritis brings the following medications to the clinic for a follow-up visit: naproxen, ibuprofen, sulindac, and digoxin. Which of the following should the nurse be certain to emphasize with the client?
    1. Clarify the purposes of each medication.
    2. Determine if she has other medications at home.
    3. Assess her for any chronic heart condition.
    4. Suggest she stop taking these medications until she sees the health care provider.

54. Correct answer - 1. The nurse must clarify with the client the purposes of each medication because the first three are all nonsteroidal anti-inflammatory medications and should not be taken at the same time. Option 2 is pertinent but not related to the medications she brought. Option 3 is not relevant to the medication review. Option 4 is not important at this time because she is at the clinic and will have a visit with the health care provider.
CN: Safe, effective care environment

55. Four hours after a client with a CVA is admitted, you assess the following: BP 170/80; apical pulse, 58 and regular; respirations, 13; axillary temperature, 101° F. What should you do next?
    1. Report these vital signs to the health care provider.
    2. Increase the frequency of vital sign assessment.
    3. Assess the client for an overdistended bladder.
    4. Assess for signs of overhydration.

55. Correct answer - 1. Brain injury can both elevate and depress blood pressure. Slow pulse, slow respirations, and increased pulse pressure are associated with CVA and may indicate increasing intracranial pressure (ICP). Option 2: Although this will, no doubt, be done, the important thing is to report these changes to the health care provider. Option 3: These vital signs are associated with increased intracranial pressure and are not a result of a distended bladder. Option 4: These are not the signs associated with fluid overload.
CN: Physiological integrity

56. A 68-year-old woman hits her head on the bathtub. On admission to the neurological unit, she has a decreased level of consciousness (LOC). Positioning orders are: head of bed (HOB) elevated; head in neutral alignment with no neck flexion or head rotation; no sharp hip flexion. What is the best rationale for this positioning order?
    1. To decrease cerebral arterial pressure.
    2. To avoid impeding venous outflow.
    3. To prevent flexion contractures.
    4. To prevent aspiration of stomach contents.

56. Correct answer - 2. Any activity or position that impedes venous outflow from the head may contribute to increased volume inside the skull and possibly increase ICP. Option 1: Cerebral arterial pressure will be affected by the balance between oxygen and carbon dioxide. Option 3: Flexion contractures are not a problem at this time. Option 4: Stomach contents can still be aspirated in this position, although it is less likely than in a flat position.
CN: Physiological integrity

57. While assessing a client immediately postop from surgery to treat a knee injury that occurred in a football game, the nurse notes bruising around the knee and understands that bruising is
    1. the result of tibial dislocation.
    2. the result of knee manipulations during surgery.
    3. referred to as a charley-horse.
    4. the sign of trauma and the inflammatory response.

57. Correct answer - 4. Bruising is caused by bleeding into the tissues from the injury. Option 1: A knee injury is not related to a tibial dislocation. Option 2: Bruising would not come from the manipulation. Option 3: A charley-horse is the pain associated with muscle pull.
    CN: Physiological integrity

58. What should the nurse know about the interaction of piperacillin/tazobactam (Zosyn) and gentamicin (Garamycin)?
    1. Mix drugs together and give by I.V. infusion.
    2. Give drugs separately, waiting 1 hour between doses.
    3. Administer drugs at same time via I.V. bolus.
    4. Drugs should be given separately, waiting 15 minutes.

58. Correct answer - 2. High doses of penicillin G and extended-spectrum penicillins, such as piperacillin/tazobactam, inactivate aminoglycosides (gentamicin). This interaction is important in clients with poor renal function because of elevated blood concentrations of both drugs. Options 1 and 3: Penicillins should not be mixed in the same I.V. fluid with aminoglycosides. Option 4: Doses of both drugs should be separated by at least 1 hour.
    CN: Physiological integrity

59. A client has had gentamicin sulfate (Garamycin), 80 mg prescribed to be given I.V. every 8 hours. Over what time period should this drug be infused?
    1. 5 minutes
    2. 10 minutes
    3. 20 minutes
    4. 30 minutes

59. Correct answer - 4. The nurse should infuse gentamicin sulfate I.V. over at least 30 minutes. Infusing the drug more rapidly may increase the client's risk of adverse reactions. Options 1, 2, and 3: These time periods are too short and may expose the client to adverse effects.
    CN: Safe, effective care environment

60. A client with Lyme disease has tetracycline hydrochloride (Achromycin), 500 mg PO q.i.d. prescribed. The nurse should teach the client to take the drug
    1. before meals on an empty stomach.
    2. with a full glass of milk.
    3. with aluminum hydroxide (Amphojel).
    4. with an iron supplement like ferris sulfate (Feosol).

60. Correct answer - 1. Tetracycline should be taken on an empty stomach because certain foods can bind with the drug, preventing its absorption. Options 2, 3, and 4: The drug should not be taken with calcium, milk, magnesium, aluminum, or iron because these substances also bind with tetracycline, inhibiting its absorption.
    CN: Health promotion and maintenance

61. A client getting an antineoplastic agent by I.V. infusion tells the nurse, "My arm is burning." Which action should the nurse take *first?*
    1. Slow the I.V. infusion.
    2. Chart the client's complaint.
    3. Call the client's health care provider.
    4. Stop the I.V. infusion.

61. Correct answer - 4. Antineoplastic agents can cause tissue sloughing and necrosis if extravasated. The infusion should be stopped immediately and the I.V. site assessed for extravasation. Option 1: The infusion should be stopped, not slowed. Option 2 is not the first action to be taken. It should be documented later. Option 3 is not the first action to be taken. Call after stopping the I.V. and assessing the site.
    CN: Physiological integrity

62. A client with generalized second- and third-degree burns has a health care provider's order for morphine 10 mg q2-3h prn for pain. The order has no administration route stipulated. The nurse questions the order, knowing that the best route for this client to achieve pain relief is
    1. orally.
    2. intravenously.
    3. intramuscularly.
    4. subcutaneously.

62. Correct answer - 2. This route provides rapid absorption. Option 1: This client should be kept NPO until his condition has stabilized. Options 3 and 4: Edema may keep the medication from being absorbed.
    CN: Safe, effective care environment

63. A 19-year-old man has praziquantel (Biltricide) prescribed for a worm infestation. While instructing the client about the drug, what should the nurse teach?
    1. Take the drug on an empty stomach.
    2. Take the drug with meals and swallow tablet whole.
    3. Keep active and exercise vigorously on treatment day.
    4. Don't give aspirin if headache occurs.

63. Correct answer - 2. This drug has a bitter taste and could cause gagging and vomiting. Option 1: The drug should be taken with food to avoid GI upset. Option 3: This drug may cause drowsiness and malaise, so heavy activity should be avoided on treatment day. Option 4: Headache is an adverse effect. There is no contraindication to aspirin.
    CN: Physiological integrity

64. The medication cimetidine (Tagamet) is given to a client with duodenal ulcer to
    1. reduce nausea and vomiting.
    2. decrease intestinal spasms.
    3. decrease acid production.
    4. increase gastric emptying.

64. Correct answer - 3. Cimetidine is one of a class of histamine-blocking drugs that decrease production of gastric actions. Options 1, 2, and 4 are not actions of cimetidine.
    CN: Safe, effective care environment

65. The key psychosocial conflict, "generativity versus stagnation," is considered vital during which developmental growth stage?
    1. Young adulthood
    2. Middle adulthood
    3. Older adulthood
    4. Elder adulthood

65. Correct answer - 2. Middle adulthood occurs between ages 35 to 65, and generativity versus stagnation is a major psychosocial variable during this phase. Option 1: The key conflict here is "intimacy versus isolation." Option 3: The key conflict here is "integrity versus despair." Option 4: There is no key developmental conflict that defines elder (85 plus years) adults.
CN: Health promotion and maintenance

66. A person's stress response is *initially* related to his
    1. adaptation to a threat.
    2. perception of a threat.
    3. hormonal responses.
    4. resistance to a stressor.

66. Correct answer - 2. Until a person perceives something as a threat, his stress response does not begin. Option 1 and 3 are later responses. Option 4 does not relate to a threat, thus there is no stress response.
CN: Physiological integrity

67. Which of the following is correct concerning hepatitis?
    1. Different forms of the disease may have similar symptoms.
    2. The virus attacks the bile ducts, causing jaundice.
    3. The virus is excreted through oral secretions.
    4. A carrier state does not exist.

67. Correct answer - 1. There are five types of viral hepatitis: A, B, C, D, and E; disease transmission varies, but similar symptoms may occur. Option 2: The virus attacks the Kupfer cells of the liver. Jaundice results from the enlarged liver compressing the bile ducts. Option 3: The virus is excreted in feces or blood serum. Option 4: Carrier states have been identified for hepatitis B, C, and possibly D.
CN: Physiological integrity

68. A client with extensive burns of the chest and neck is at risk for atelectasis because of
    1. pulmonary edema.
    2. decreased alveolar surfactant.
    3. pressure of burn dressings on thorax.
    4. insufficient fluid replacement.

68. Correct answer - 2. Alveoli are kept open with surfactant, which is diminished from smoke inhalation and damage to respiratory mucosa. Option 1 could occur if there was fluid volume overload. Option 3: Dressings are not commonly used in burns and would not cause atelectasis. Option 4 could cause hypovolemic shock, not atelectasis.
CN: Physiological integrity

69. A client with malignant melanoma is being discharged after surgery to remove the tumor. To prevent recurrence of this tumor, during discharge teaching the nurse emphasizes
    1. proper care of the wound.
    2. use of sunscreens and hats.
    3. how to do range of motion exercises.
    4. eating a diet high in vitamins A, B, and C.

69. Correct answer - 2. Reducing exposure to the sun and use of sunscreens is a major teaching strategy to prevent recurrence of this type of cancer. Options 1, 3, and 4 do not prevent recurrence, but should be included in teaching, if appropriate.
CN: Safe, effective care environment

70. A client is 5 hours postoperative after a hip replacement. The nurse should position the client's affected leg in which position?
    1. External rotation
    2. Abduction
    3. Flexion
    4. Hyperextension

70. Correct answer - 2. A client who has had a hip replacement should have an abduction pillow placed between his legs to separate them. Options 1, 3, and 4 are harmful positions because they could dislodge the prosthesis.
CN: Physiological integrity

71. A client comes to the emergency department with an inversion ankle sprain. Such a sprain occurs when the
    1. foot is turned outward.
    2. person is flat footed.
    3. foot is twisted inward.
    4. foot is stretched downward.

71. Correct answer - 3. An inversion sprain occurs when the foot is turned inward (remember in/in). Option 1 refers to an eversion sprain (remember evert = turned outward). Option 2: This sprain happens to persons with high arches. Option 4 has no effect on an inversion sprain.
CN: Physiological integrity

72. A client is receiving a continuous I.V. infusion of milrinone lactate (Primacor). The nurse explains that he should know that this drug
    1. does not require a loading dose.
    2. produces vasoconstriction.
    3. is typically given with digoxin and diuretics.
    4. may cause hypertension.

72. Correct answer - 3. Milrinone lactate is typically given with digoxin and diuretics to treat acute heart failure. Option 1: The drug does require an initial loading dose of 50 mcg/kg I.V., administered over 10 minutes. Option 2: The drug causes vasodilation by directly relaxing vascular smooth muscle. Option 4: Hypertension is not a known adverse effect of milrinone.
CN: Physiological integrity

73. The primary substance associated with metabolic acidosis is
    1. hydrogen.
    2. bicarbonate ion.
    3. carbonic acid.
    4. carbon dioxide.

73. Correct answer - 2. Metabolic acidosis is associated with the kidneys and bicarbonate. Option 1 may be excreted in metabolic acidosis or used to make more bicarbonate (HCO_3). Options 3 and 4 are primary substances in respiratory acidosis.
CN: Physiological integrity

74. Following surgery on his left leg, a client is to be up with crutches and touchdown weight-bearing. Which comment by a client being taught crutch walking with touch-down weight-bearing *best* identifies the need for more teaching?
    1. "I need to use both crutches while walking."
    2. "I will move my right foot forward before the left one when walking."
    3. "I'll put all of my weight on my right foot as I step forward."
    4. "I'll use the crutches to go up and down stairs."

74. Correct answer - 3. Touchdown weight-bearing means that the client can put 25 pounds of weight on his left leg so he won't put all his weight on his right leg. Options 1, 2, and 4 are correct statements.
CN: Safe, effective care environment

75. While assessing the fingertips of a client with Raynaud phenomenon, the nurse understands that the color changes proceed from
    1. white to blue to red.
    2. blue to red to white.
    3. red to white to blue.
    4. white to red to blue.

75. Correct answer - 4. Blanching followed by redness then cyanosis occurs in Raynaud phenomenon because of the arterial spasms and venous stasis. Options 1 2, and 3 are incorrect patterns.
CN: Physiological integrity

76. A 45-year-old female has acute cholecystitis. She should be taught to avoid which foods to lessen painful gallbladder attacks?
    1. Scalloped potatoes
    2. Baked ham with gravy
    3. Macaroni with tomato sauce
    4. Cottage cheese and pineapple salad

76. Correct answer - 2. Ham and gravy should be avoided as they are high in fat and can precipitate an attack. Option 1: Scalloped potatoes have less fat per serving than the ham and gravy. Options 3 and 4: These are foods that are low in fat and may be taken without causing attacks.
CN: Physiological integrity

77. A nurse recently exposed to hepatitis A may be given which substance to lessen chance of active infection?
    1. Human serum albumin
    2. Hepatitis B vaccine
    3. Immune serum globulin
    4. High doses of vitamins B and C

77. Correct answer - 3. Administration of immune serum globu-lin should prevent an active infection, if given soon after exposure. Options 2, 3, and 4 are incorrect as they don't affect hepatitis A transmission.
CN: Safe, effective care environment

78. The highest risk of developing osteoporosis is
found in
    1. obese women.
    2. African-American women.
    3. women who smoke cigarettes.
    4. postmenopausal women.

78. Correct answer - 4. Postmenopausal women
have the highest risk of developing
osteoporosis. Option 1: Obesity does not
increase the risk of osteoporosis. Option 2:
Osteoporosis is more common in white and
Asian individuals than women in other groups.
Option 3: There is an increased risk in those
individuals who have experienced chronic
malnutrition and those who smoke .
CN: Health promotion and maintenance.

79. The drug of choice for pancreatic pain control
is
    1. meperidine.
    2. pentazocine.
    3. morphine.
    4. propantheline.

79. Correct answer - 1. Meperidine is the drug of
choice for pancreatic pain. Option 2:
Pentazocine is an alternative for clients who can
not tolerate meperidine. Option 3: Morphine
usually is avoided because it's associated with
spasm of the ampulla of Vater. Option 4:
Propantheline is a parenteral anticholinergic
drug that may be ordered to decrease vagal
stimulation and inhibit pancreatic enzyme
secretion.
CN: Physiological integrity

80. A nurse caring for a client with a duodenal
ulcer understands that the client's pain episodes
    1. occur when the duodenum is empty.
    2. are usually constant and burning.
    3. are localized on the left side of the
umbilicus.
    4. result from the presence of pancreatic juice
in the duodenum.

80. Correct answer - 1. Pain often occurs at night
when the upper GI system is empty. Options 2,
3, and 4: Duodenal ulcer pain is right epigastric
to the right of the umbilicus, not the left. It is
caused by the highly acid chyme from the
stomach into the duodenum, not pancreatic
secretions.
CN: Physiological integrity

81. A client who is in respiratory failure as a result
of acute pulmonary edema is placed on a
mechanical ventilator. The *primary* goal of
mechanical ventilation in the treatment of acute
pulmonary edema is to
    1. facilitate the removal of oropharyngeal
secretions.
    2. monitor mean pulmonary artery pressure.
    3. administer concentrations of oxygen under
pressure.
    4. increase venous return to the heart.

81. Correct answer - 3. Mechanical ventilation is
required if respiratory failure occurs despite
optimal management in pulmonary edema. The
use of positive end expiratory pressure (PEEP)
is more effective in improving oxygenation than
other methods such as nasal cannulas in this
situation. Options 1, 2, and 4: Oropharyngeal
secretions may be removed by suctioning
and/or diuretics; mean pulmonary artery
pressure is monitored by a pulmonary artery
catheter. A mechanical ventilator would *reduce*
venous return, not increase it.
CN: Physiological integrity

82. A client is admitted to the hospital in acute pulmonary edema. The client is tachypneic and dyspneic. The client should be placed in which of these positions?
    1. Trendelenburg
    2. Supine
    3. Right side-lying
    4. High-Fowler's

83. A client who has angina pectoris is given instructions about the use of nitroglycerin ointment (Nitro-Bid). The client requires *further* instructions if he makes which of these comments?
    1. "Every time I apply the drug, I'll change the site where I put it."
    2. "I'll store the drug container in a cool place."
    3. "If I get ringing in my ears, I'll remove the patch right away."
    4. "After I put the right amount of the drug on the patch, I'll put it on a non-hairy skin surface."

84. A client who is receiving digoxin (Lanoxin) should be observed for early adverse effects, which include
    1. anorexia.
    2. tachycardia.
    3. dyskinesia.
    4. constipation.

85. On the second postoperative day, a client's wound appeared slightly swollen and inflamed. These assessment findings are
    1. normal at this time.
    2. signs of a beginning infection.
    3. signs of collagen deposition.
    4. signs of the wound's maturation phase.

82. Correct answer - 4. High-Fowler's position has the immediate effect of decreasing venous return, lowering the output of the right ventricle, and decreasing lung congestion (i.e., reducing preload). All of these effects improve respiratory functioning. Options 1, 2, and 3: These positions would increase venous return and right ventricular output (preload), which would favor the reabsorption of edema fluid in the lungs. This, in turn, would make the client's breathing more labored.
CN: Physiological integrity

83. Correct answer - 3. Although nitroglycerin has several adverse effects (i.e., headache, postural hypotension, circulatory collapse) ringing in the ears (tinnitus) is not one of them. Options 1, 2, and 4 are all correct answers, indicating that the client has understood the instructions. Rotating the site on a non-hairy skin surface and storing the medication in a cool place are all recommended.
CN: Physiological integrity

84. Correct answer - 1. Anorexia is an early adverse effect of digitalis. Options 2, 3, and 4: Bradycardia (rather than tachycardia), muscle weakness (rather than dyskinesia), and diarrhea (rather than constipation), are other adverse effects of digitalis.
CN: Physiological integrity

85. Correct answer - 1. These are normal findings in the initial healing phase. Option 2: These findings may be signs of a beginning infection at a later point in the healing process. Options 3 and 4 are wrong for this time period.
CN: Physiological integrity

86. The teaching plan for a client who is scheduled for a cardiac catheterization should include which of the following information?
    1. The client will be kept NPO for 2 hours before the procedure.
    2. An indwelling urinary catheter will be inserted into the client immediately prior to the procedure.
    3. The client may experience a flushed feeling when the contrast dye is injected during the procedure.
    4. A mild cathartic will be given to the client after the procedure.

86. Correct answer - 3. One fairly common adverse effect of contrast dye (i.e., iohexol injection [Omnipaque 350]) is flushing. Another relatively common sensation the client may feel during the procedure is palpitation, which may occur when catheter tip touches the myocardium. Options 1, 2, and 4: The client is kept NPO for 8 to 12 hours before the test and does not require an indwelling urinary catheter or cathartic.
CN: Safe, effective care environment

87. A client is admitted to the hospital after a spinal cord injury. Following further evaluation, he is diagnosed as having a partial transection of the spinal cord at the level of the fifth cervical vertebra. He is quadriplegic. Several weeks later he develops autonomic hyperreflexia (autonomic dysreflexia). Which of these actions should the nurse take *first?*
    1. Place the client in a sitting position.
    2. Passively exercise his extremities every 2 hours.
    3. Get an order for a stat dose of hydralazine hydrochloride (Apresoline).
    4. Notify the health care provider.

87. Correct answer - 1. Autonomic hyperreflexia (autonomic dysreflexia) is a medical emergency that generally happens after spinal shock has subsided in clients who have had cord injuries above the level of the sixth thoracic vertebra. It occurs as a result of exaggerated autonomic responses to stimuli that are innocuous in normal individuals, (i.e., distended bladder or bowel, draft of cold air). In this situation, the first step is to place the client in a sitting position to lower his blood pressure, then to determine and remove the stimuli that have triggered the condition. Options 2, 3, and 4: Exercising the client's extremities will not help in this emergency situation, and in fact may aggravate it; Apresoline is sometimes given I.V. when initial measures (i.e., sitting client upright and attempting to remove the triggering stimuli) are ineffective; and the health care provider should be notified, but only after initial measures are taken.
CN: Physiological integrity

88. A nurse has given a client instructions in preparation for an electroencephalogram. The client has understood the instructions if he makes which of these statements?
    1. "I can't eat or drink anything for 8 hours before the test."
    2. "Electrodes will be attached to my scalp just before the test."
    3. "A contrast medium will be injected into my veins during the test."
    4. "The color of my urine will change for a few hours after the test."

88. Correct answer - 2. For electroencephalogram, electrodes are arranged on the scalp to record the electrical activity in various regions of the head. Options 1, 2, and 4: Although the client will be instructed to avoid stimulants (i.e., coffee, cocoa, tea, cola) prior to the test, he can eat because an altered blood glucose level can cause changes in the brain wave pattern. This is a non-invasive procedure, so a contrast medium is not given, nor should the color of the client's urine change.
CN: Safe, effective care environment

89. A client is admitted to the hospital because he had a grand mal seizure. The nurse should include which of these notations on his care plan?
    1. "Keep in a chest restraint at all times."
    2. "Pad the side rails of bed."
    3. "Maintain in high-Fowler's position."
    4. "Have endotracheal tube at bedside."

89. Correct answer - 2. Protecting the client's safety is critically important. One way to do this is to pad the side rails of the bed in case the client should have a seizure. Options 1, 3, and 4: No restraints should be used in the event that the client has a seizure. There is no reason to maintain the client in high-Fowler's position or to have an endotracheal tube at the bedside.
CN: Safe, effective care environment

90. A client has been hospitalized for 3 weeks because he sustained a compound fracture of the third and fourth lumbar vertebrae, which resulted in the complete transection of his spinal cord. He has been on bedrest since admission to the hospital. It would be *essential* that the nurse make which of these assessments of the client periodically?
    1. Rate and quality of pedal pulses
    2. Presence of Homan's signs
    3. Ability to move his lower extremities
    4. Pressure on his skin, especially bony areas

90. Correct answer - 4. A client who has a complete transection of the spinal cord at the third and fourth lumbar vertebrae will be a paraplegic. As a result, he probably will be unable to move or change his position by himself. Therefore, he is at risk for developing pressure ulcers, which require frequent assessment. Options 1, 2, and 3: Note that the stem of the item asks you to select an "essential" assessment, or to prioritize your assessments. Because the client lost the ability to move or feel sensation in his lower extremities, checking him for movement or the pain associated with Homan's sign is not critical. The rate and quality of his pedal pulses is not as important as checking him for pressure areas.
CN: Physiological integrity

91. A client has recently been diagnosed as having Parkinson's disease. Because of his diagnosis, his care plan would most likely include which of these nursing diagnoses?
    1. Perceptual alteration related to photophobia.
    2. Bathing self-care deficit related to muscle spasticity.
    3. Alteration in thought processes related to intellectual impairment.
    4. Impaired written communication related to hand tremor.

92. A client is to have arterial blood gases (ABGs) drawn from the radial artery. Prior to drawing the ABGs, it would be *most* important to make which of these assessments of the selected extremity?
    1. Response to the Allen test.
    2. Skin temperature in the radial pulse area.
    3. Results of the capillary filling time.
    4. Strength and rhythm of the radial pulse.

93. A client is being prepared for a bronchoscopy. Which of the following information should he be given about the test?
    1. Several sputum specimens will be collected before the test.
    2. Allergies to dyes will be determined before the test.
    3. Coughing is to be avoided for several hours after the test.
    4. Drinking and eating should be avoided until the gag reflex returns after the test.

91. Correct answer - 4. One of the early signs of Parkinson's disease is tremors of the hands, which affects handwriting by making it get smaller, particularly towards the end of words (micrographia). Options 1, 2, and 3: In Parkinson's disease, eye problems are related to the loss of autonomic movements (i.e., blinking) rather than photophobia; the muscles are rigid, rather than spastic; and intellectual impairment does not occur in the majority of clients.
CN: Physiological integrity

92. Correct answer - 1. Collateral circulation to the area must be confirmed before the blood is drawn. Capillary filling time is used to assess arterial flow to the extremities. If no collateral circulation existed and the artery became occluded, ischemia and infection to the area distal to the site could occur. Collateral circulation is checked by the Allen test for the radial and ulnar arteries or by an ultrasonic Doppler test for all arteries used, including the femoral and brachial. Options 2, 3, and 4: None of these will evaluate collateral circulation.
CN: Safe, effective care environment

93. Correct answer - 4. During the test, the client's nasal pharynx and oral pharynx are anesthetized, which affects his ability to swallow. Thus, the presence of the gag reflex needs to be determined before oral intake is allowed to avoid aspiration. Options 1, 2, and 3: There is no need to collect sputum specimens for a bronchoscopy or to determine if the client has allergies to dyes because a contrast medium will not be given. Although the client may not be able to cough in the initial period after the test because his throat has been anesthetized, coughing should be encouraged as soon as possible.
CN: Safe, effective care environment

94. A client who has advanced chronic airflow limitation is observed for symptoms of cor pulmonale, which include
    1. dry, hacking cough and diaphoresis.
    2. blood-tinged sputum and orthopnea.
    3. distended neck veins and ascites.
    4. paroxysmal nocturnal dyspnea and rales.

95. An electrocardiogram (ECG) is ordered for a client who is thought to have myocardial ischemia. If he does, the nurse should expect to see ECG changes in the ST segment and which of these waves?
    1. P
    2. S
    3. T
    4. U

96. A client is returned to the unit following a hiatal hernia repair. In the immediate postoperative period, the *priority* nursing diagnosis should be
    1. pain related to surgical procedure.
    2. impaired gas exchange related to general anesthesia.
    3. risk for fluid volume deficit related to being NPO.
    4. impaired physical mobility related to operative site discomfort.

97. What is the most important goal of preoperative teaching for a client scheduled for surgery?
    1. Explain the informed consent policy.
    2. Prepare the client for anesthesia.
    3. Reduce the client's anxiety.
    4. Discuss the required preoperative diagnostic tests.

94. Correct answer - 3. Symptoms of cor pulmonale are related to the dilation and failure of the right ventricle with subsequent intravascular volume expansion and systemic venous congestion. Thus, the symptoms are caused by right-sided heart failure. Options 1, 2, and 4: All of these symptoms are associated with left-sided heart failure.
CN: Physiological integrity

95. Correct answer - 3. Myocardial ischemia causes the T wave to be larger and inverted because of altered late repolarization. Options 1, 3, and 4 are incorrect answers.
CN: Physiological integrity

96. Correct answer - 2. In the immediate postop period, impaired gas exchange is the major concern because of diaphragmatic repair and the client's hesitancy to deep breathe. Options 1, 3, and 4 are possible post nursing diagnoses but do not have the priority of impaired gas exchange.
CN: Safe, effective care environment

97. Correct answer - 3. Reducing anxiety over a medical procedure minimizes postoperative complications, shortens the recovery period, and increases client compliance with treatments. Options 1, 2, and 4 are appropriate preoperative teachings that contribute to the goal of reducing anxiety.
CN: Physiological integrity

98. What is the *best* nursing intervention for a postoperative client who has a nursing diagnosis of impaired gas exchange?
    1. Administer antibiotics to prevent pneumonia.
    2. Teach upper body range of motion exercises.
    3. Administer oxygen via nasal cannula for 24 hours postoperatively.
    4. Encourage use of an incentive spirometer.

98. Correct answer - 4. Use of an incentive spirometer helps the client fully expand the lungs to improve gas exchange. Option 1 is a medical intervention carried out by the nurse. Option 2 is done later, but is not to enhance gas exchange. Option 3 may be used but does not contribute to deep breathing and lung expansion.
CN: Physiological integrity

99. A client is in the emergency department complaining of chest pain with a diagnosis of possible MI. When checking his cardiac rhythm on a cardiac monitor, the nurse observes eight multifocal premature ventricular contractions (PVCs) in a minute strip. Which of these actions should the nurse take *next?*
    1. Change the client's electrocardiogram leads.
    2. Get an order for an antiarrhythmic drug.
    3. Ask the client to change his position.
    4. Continue to evaluate the client's condition frequently.

99. Correct answer - 2. In the client with an acute MI, PVCs are considered serious precursors of ventricular tachycardia and ventricular fibrillation when they (1) occur in increasing number, more than six per minute; (2) are multi-focal or originate from several areas in the heart; (3) occur in pairs or triplets; and (4) occur in the vulnerable phase of conduction. To decrease myocardial irritability, the cause must be determined and, if possible, corrected. An antiarrhythmic drug may be used for immediate and possibly long-term therapy. Thus, the nurse should check the hospital's protocol for administering an antiarrhythmic like lidocaine hydrochloride. Options 1, 3, and 4: None of these actions will help to correct this life-threatening situation.
CN: Physiological integrity

100. What is the *most* important point that the nurse should stress when teaching nursing assistants about avoiding infections?
    1. Avoid respiratory pathogens.
    2. Use correct handwashing techniques.
    3. Maintain nutritional health.
    4. Use aseptic technique for wound care.

100. Correct answer - 2. Correct and frequent handwashing prevents transmission of infection. Options 1, 3, and 4 are more important in healing current infections.
CN: Health promotion and maintenance

101. A client with regional ileitis (Chron's disease) has a history of diarrhea and weight loss. When doing an assessment, what would the nurse expect the client to report about the diarrhea episodes?
    1. She has frequent, bloody stools.
    2. Her stools contains pus and blood.
    3. Her stools are watery and contain mucus.
    4. Her stools are foul-smelling, with fat molecules in them.

101. Correct answer - 4. This is the classic description of the diarrhea of regional ileitis. Options 1, 2, and 3 all are characteristic of the diarrhea of ulcerative colitis.
CN: Physiological integrity

102. A client who just had a colonoscopy complains of severe gas pain. The nurse should explain that the gas pains are
    1. common after a colonoscopy.
    2. a sign of a possible complication.
    3. a sign that the colon's function has returned.
    4. eased with deep breathing.

102. Correct answer - 1. Because the colon is distended with gas (carbon dioxide) for better visualization, gas pains are common and are not a complication. Option 2: Abdominal gas after a colonoscopy is a normal finding, not a sign of a complication. Gas pains may not be a sign that the colon's function has returned (option 3), but may be a sign of ileus. Option 4: This has little relationship to gas pain relief.
CN: Physiological integrity

103. A client is ready for discharge following a small bowel resection for regional ileitis. When teaching the client self-care at home, the nurse should include which information?
    1. The surgery should cure her regional ileitis.
    2. Her symptoms may recur at a later date.
    3. Stress has no relationship to her condition.
    4. She should maintain her low-roughage diet.

103. Correct answer - 2. Regional ileitis can recur as other intestinal areas become inflamed. Options 1, 3, and 4 are not true statements about regional ileitis.
CN: Safe, effective care environment

104. Common adverse effects of morphine include
    1. diarrhea and abdominal flatulence.
    2. headache and mydriasis.
    3. nausea and abdominal flatulence.
    4. constipation and urine retention.

104. Correct answer - 4. These are two very common adverse effects. Options 1, 2, and 3 are not adverse effects of morphine.
CN: Safe, effective care environment

105. A 39-year-old firefighter is hospitalized with deep, partial-thickness burns over his chest, arms, and neck. He is in severe pain and requests narcotics every time a nurse enters his room. The nurse knows that his requests for pain medication are related to his
    1. previous use of narcotic analgesics.
    2. fear of achieving poor pain relief.
    3. exposed nerve endings in burned areas.
    4. desire to forget his harrowing experiences.

105. Correct answer - 3. Deep second-degree (partial-thickness) burns expose nerve endings in the dermis, causing severe pain. Options 1 and 2 may or may not have relevance to his current condition. Option 4 may have some relevance but is not treated with narcotic analgesics.
CN: Physiological integrity

106. I.V. fluid replacement for a client with extensive second- and third-degree burns includes lactated Ringer's solution and colloids. What should be the amount of fluids given I.V., according to replacement formulas?
    1. ¼ total amount of fluid in first 8 hours, then ½ and ¼ in second and third 8 hours, respectively.
    2. ¼ total amount in first 8 hours, then ¼ and ½ in second and third 8 hours, respectively.
    3. ½ total amount in first 8 hours, then ¼ each in second and third 8 hours.
    4. ¼ total amount in first 8 hours and ½ in second and third 8 hours.

106. Correct answer - 3. The major fluid replacement should be in first 8 hours to replace fluids lost from the vascular compartment to interstitial tissues to prevent hypovolemic shock. Options 1, 2, and 4 are incorrect replacement schedules.
CN: Safe, effective care environment

107. A client has an order for 12 mg of morphine sulfate. The morphine comes supplied as 15 mg/ ml. What is the correct amount of solution to administer?
    1. 1.25 ml
    2. 0.8 ml
    3. 0.6 ml
    4. 1.5 ml

107. Correct answer - 2. This ratio is [15 mg/1 ml = 12 mg/x (ml)], thus x = 0.8 ml.
CN: Safe, effective care environment

108. A client is 2 days postoperative after abdominal surgery. Which finding by the nurse would indicate the client has a postoperative complication?
    1. Low-grade temperature.
    2. Weakness when ambulating.
    3. Abdominal distention.
    4. Muscle soreness.

108. Correct answer - 3. Postoperative persistent abdominal distention may indicate paralytic ileus. Options 1, 2, and 4 are expected outcomes following surgery.
CN: Physiological integrity

109. What are the *best* nursing interventions to prevent bleeding from esophageal varices?
1. Increasing fluid intake to prevent esophageal drying.
2. Encouraging dietary intake of high fiber foods to prevent constipation and straining.
3. Encouraging isometric exercises at least three times daily to prevent muscle wasting.
4. Teaching to avoid use of aspirin and aspirin-like medications.

109. Correct answer - 4. These medications may increase chance of bleeding from varices. Options 1 and 2: Fluid intake is limited, and foods are to be low fiber to prevent excoriation of varices. Option 3: Isometric exercise increase intra-abdominal pressure, which could lead to rupture of varices. They are therefore contraindicated.
CN: Physiological integrity

110. A 55-year-old male has a bowel obstruction and is being treated with an intestinal tube connected to wall suction. What is the *most* important nursing intervention while the client has the intestinal tube in place?
1. Measuring abdominal girth every 12 hours.
2. Turning client side to side as prescribed.
3. Providing sips of water to facilitate passing the tube through the bowel.
4. Putting antacids into the intestinal tube to lessen bowel reaction.

110. Correct answer - 2. Turning side to side helps the intestinal tube's passage to site of obstruction. Option 1: Abdominal girth should be measured q2-4h to note distention. Options 3 and 4: The client should be kept NPO with I.V. fluid therapy.
CN: Safe, effective care environment

111. A client has a bowel obstruction caused by adhesions from surgery several years ago. While being treated with an intestinal tube, he develops hypotension. The nurse initiates interventions knowing the hypotension is most likely due to
1. septicemia.
2. hypokalemia.
3. hyponatremia.
4. weight loss.

111. Correct answer - 1. Bowel obstruction may lead to abdominal infection and septicemia. Options 2, 3, and 4 may be associated with bowel obstruction but don't result in septicemia and hypotension.
CN: Physiological integrity

112. While doing a physical examination on a client with an elbow injury, the nurse notes crepitus in the elbow joint. This finding is a
1. normal finding.
2. result of ligament damage.
3. noisy sound in a joint.
4. tenderness around a joint.

112. Correct answer - 3. Crepitus refers to a noisy or cracking sound in a joint. Options 1 and 2: It is not a normal finding, nor is it a result of ligament damage. It is usually related to arthritis. Option 4: Crepitus does not cause tenderness around a joint.
CN: Physiological integrity

113. A client comes to the emergency department short of breath; he cannot speak because of severe dyspnea. He has a history of an MI and several episodes of heart failure. When auscultating his chest, what would the nurse expect to hear?
    1. A friction rub and clear breath sounds.
    2. A murmur and crackles.
    3. A friction rub and crackles.
    4. An S_3 gallop and crackles.

113. Correct answer - 4. An S_3 gallop is characteristic of heart failure; crackles indicate the presence of intra-alveolar fluid, which may result from left-sided heart failure. Option 1: This client would not have clear breath sounds. Option 2: Heart failure does not cause a murmur. Option 3: Pleurisy, not heart failure, causes a friction rub.
CN: Physiological integrity

114. What is the *first* action the nurse should take when entering the room of a client who is having generalized seizure?
    1. Insert a padded tongue blade into the client's mouth.
    2. Turn the client's head to the side.
    3. Put the siderails down to prevent injury.
    4. Call a code.

114. Correct answer - 2. During a generalized seizure, the client's head should be turned to the side to let secretions drain and his airway open. After the seizure, he may be placed on his side. Option 1: During a seizure, the jaw is clenched. The nurse should never force the jaw open to insert objects. Option 3: Siderails should remain up to prevent further injury. Option 4: Codes are called for clients in cardiac arrest.
CN: Safe, effective care environment

115. A client with acute glomerulonephritis tells the nurse he has been drinking more water because he knows it is important to do so when one has an infection. What is the *best* response?
    1. "That's good, I'm glad you are interested in doing what is good for you."
    2. "Fruit juices would be better for you; what kind of juice do you like?"
    3. "Didn't your health care provider tell you that you cannot drink anything?"
    4. "With most infections, drinking a lot of fluids is good, but in this situation, your fluid intake must be restricted."

115. Correct answer - 4. In clients with glomerulonephritis, fluid intake must be restricted to equal fluid output to ensure that fluid is not retained while kidney function is impaired. Options 1 and 2 do not convey the importance of restricting fluids. Option 3: Total restrictions of fluids is not necessary.
CN: Physiological integrity

116. Which statement made by a client beginning hemodialysis shows he understands the treatment?
    1. "I will feel better immediately after dialysis."
    2. "I can eat and drink whatever I want because I'm on dialysis."
    3. "Dialysis is a complication-free procedure."
    4. "The dialysis takes about 4 hours and must be done 3 days a week."

116. Correct answer - 4. Hemodialysis usually takes 3 to 5 hours and is done three times a week. Option 1: Most clients feel best the day after dialysis. Option 2: Protein, sodium, and potassium usually are restricted, and calories and carbohydrates are increased. Fluids are restricted. Option 3: Complications can occur.
CN: Health promotion and maintenance

117. The nurse is preparing a teaching plan that will be used for clients with hyperthyroidism. What should be included in this plan?
    1. Increase the room temperature if feeling cold.
    2. Eat a high-calorie, high-protein, high-carbohydrate diet.
    3. Add fiber to the diet.
    4. Use over-the-counter laxatives, as needed.

117. Correct answer - 2. Metabolism is increased in clients with hyperthyroidism. Therefore, weight loss will occur if intake is not greatly increased. Options 1, 3, and 4 are interventions for clients with hypothyroidism.
CN: Health promotion and maintenance

118. A client who is being tested for tuberculosis (TB) has a positive Mantoux result, a negative chest X-ray, and no clinical symptoms. The health care provider orders 300 mg of isoniazid daily for preventive therapy. The nurse should explain to the client that the isoniazid
    1. should be taken daily for 9 to 12 months to prevent active disease.
    2. should be taken until the Mantoux skin test reverts to normal.
    3. produces no serious adverse effects.
    4. provides active immunity to the disease as long as it is taken.

118. Correct answer - 1. Isoniazid is a bactericidal agent that stops the growth of the TB bacilli. It should be taken long-term (9 to 12 months) to prevent the disease. Option 2: Mantoux skin tests remain positive for years as long as living bacilli remain in the body. Option 3: Serious adverse effects of isoniazid include neuritis and hepatitis, which require continued evaluation. Option 4: Isoniazid does not provide active immunity; it is a bactericidal agent that inhibits growth of the bacilli.
CN: Safe, effective care environment

119. The nurse who elicits a positive Chvostek's sign would suspect that the client has which condition?
    1. Hyperkalemia
    2. Hypocalcemia
    3. Hypercalcemia
    4. Hypernatremia

119. Correct answer - 2. A positive Chvostek's sign (contraction of facial muscles when the facial nerve is tapped) indicates neuromuscular irritability, a sign of hypocalcemia.
CN: Physiological integrity

120. The nurse is caring for a client who is oliguric and who is prescribed potassium chloride 40 mEq I.V. in 1,000 ml D_5W. The nurse should question the order for the I.V. fluid because of the potential danger to the client's
    1. cardiac function.
    2. respiratory function.
    3. renal function.
    4. brain function.

120. Correct answer - 1. If the client's kidneys were not functioning, the level of potassium would increase in the bloodstream. This would adversely affect the heart muscle, causing flaccidity, arrhythmias, and cardiac arrest. Option 2: The electrolyte potassium affects the respiratory system by weakening the muscles of respiration. However, the first organ affected would be the heart. Option 3: As potassium builds, the kidneys would be unable to excrete it. However, potassium itself does not damage the tubules directly. Option 4: Potassium elevation causes a deficit in neuromuscular function. Skeletal muscles may be weak, and paresthesias of the face and tongue may occur. However, the brain would not be affected unless an acidotic condition were causing the increased potassium level.
CN: Physiological integrity

121. A male client has been admitted to the hospital to rule out an acute MI. The cardiac enzyme tests reveal a normal LDH and an elevated CPK-MB. The nurse enters the client's room and finds him pacing the floor. Which statement by the nurse would be most appropriate in this situation?
    1. "You've had a heart attack. Get back in bed."
    2. "You seem upset. Why don't you get into bed and, if you wish, we can talk for a while."
    3. "You sure have a lot of energy. Do you want to play cards?
    4. "Your health care provider doesn't want you up. Would you please get back into your bed?"

121. Correct answer - 2. Given the laboratory data, especially the elevated CPK-MB level, the nurse should realize that the client probably had a MI and that he needs to lie down and rest his heart. However, the nurse also should realize the need to respond to the client's emotional distress by acknowledging his feelings and offering to discuss his situation. Option 1: Telling the client that he had a heart attack would be giving a medical diagnosis, which has not yet been made and which would be practicing outside the scope of nursing. Option 3: This statement acknowledges the client's pacing but not his underlying concerns. Option 4: This statement tries to impose authority to control the client's behavior. It does not acknowledge his distress.
CN: Psychosocial integrity

122. When a client is diagnosed with essential hypertension, the mean arterial pressure (MAP) is used to establish blood pressure goals and evaluate treatment. Which formula is best for calculating the mean arterial pressure?
    1. MAP = diastolic blood pressure $+ \frac{1}{3}$ pulse pressure.
    2. MAP = systolic blood pressure - diastolic pressure.
    3. MAP = diastolic blood pressure $+ \frac{1}{4}$ apical pulse.
    4. MAP = systolic blood pressure + diastolic blood pressure.

122. Correct answer - 1. The ideal MAP is equal to or less than 100 mm Hg. The formula is correct as shown in the option. Option 2: The systolic blood pressure minus the diastolic blood pressure equals the pulse pressure. Option 3 and 4: These calculations are false.
CN: Physiological integrity

123. A 50-year-old man is in the same-day-surgery recovery after repair of an inguinal hernia. He is alert and taking fluids well. He feels the need to void and has tried using the urinal twice without success. He is anxious to be discharged soon. Which action should the nurse take?
    1. Help the client stand and use the urinal or toilet.
    2. Get an order to increase the client's I.V. fluids.
    3. Check the client's chart to see whether he has had voiding difficulties in the past.
    4. Withhold pain medication until the client voids.

123. Correct answer - 1. Difficulty voiding is a common problem that is easily managed by helping the client stand and void. This client is alert and planning discharge, so he can be helped to stand without endangering his condition. Option 2: The client is taking oral fluids, which can be increased if necessary. Option 3: The client is alert and can communicate if he has had prior difficulty with voiding. Option 4: Pain medication should not be withheld because the client should remain as comfortable as possible during the postoperative period.
CN: Physiological integrity

124. The nurse is preparing a client for discharge after a permanent colostomy. The discharge instructions indicate that the client will irrigate the colostomy at home. Which statement by the client indicates that teaching about the irrigation has been effective?
    1. "I'll use sterile water for the irrigation."
    2. "I'll hang the irrigation bag from the shower curtain rod, which is about 1 foot above my head."
    3. "I'll put some cloth over the stoma after the irrigation."
    4. "I'll use about a quart of warm water for irrigation."

124. Correct answer - 4. About 1,000 ml of tap water that is 100° to 105° F (37.8° to 40.5° C) is recommended for a colostomy irrigation. Irrigate gently until evacuation begins. Option 1: Sterile water is unnecessary. Option 2: The bottom of the irrigation bag should be at the client's shoulder level. If the bag is higher, the solution will enter the bowel too rapidly. Option 3: The client can expect drainage from the stoma for an hour after the irrigation, so he will need to stay in the bathroom or cover the stoma with a pouch while all the returns are eliminated.
CN: Health promotion and maintenance

125. A 21-year-old female client has recently been diagnosed with Type 1 diabetes. She is receiving 5 units of regular insulin and 15 units of NPH insulin every morning before breakfast at 7 a.m. Which statement regarding her insulin is correct?
    1. The regular insulin will begin to act rapidly (within 30 to 60 minutes) and peak in 8 hours.
    2. The NPH insulin will begin to act in 1 to $1^1/_2$ hours and will peak in 4 to 12 hours (by mid-afternoon).
    3. The regular insulin will begin to act in 1 to $1^1/_2$ hours and will peak in 5 hours (at about lunchtime).
    4. The NPH insulin will begin to act in 4 to 8 hours and will peak in 18 hours (by early evening).

125. Correct answer - 2. NPH insulin has an onset of 1 to $1^1/_2$ hours and peaks in 6 to 8 hours. Regular insulin has an onset of 30 minutes to 1 hour and peaks in $2^1/_2$ to 5 hours. Option 1: Regular insulin peakes in $2^1/_2$ to 5 hours. Option 3: Regular insulin has an onset of 30 minutes to 1 hour. Option 4: NPH insulin has an onset of 1 to $1^1/_2$ hours and peaks in 6 to 8 hours.
CN: Physiological integrity

126. A nurse asks you how chloramphenicol (Chloromycetin), which has been prescribed for one of her clients, destroys the microorganisms. Which response is the *most* accurate?
    1. It prevents synthesis of the bacterial mucopeptide.
    2. It prevents protein metabolism in bacteria that are sensitive to the drug.
    3. It binds to enzymes on the surface of bacteria sensitive to the drug.
    4. It ruptures the bacteria by increasing intracellular pressure.

126. Correct answer: 2. Chloramphenicol inhibits protein synthesis in bacteria that are susceptible to them. Option 1: The drug is not known to inhibit mucopeptide synthesis. Option 3: The drug causes plasma-mediated acetylation, not binding to bacterial enzymes. Option 4: This drug does not cause any intracellular pressure changes.
CN: Safe, effective care environment

127. A 72-year-old male client has vascular disease. Which nursing intervention would be appropriate?
    1. Encourage him to avoid caffeine and nicotine.
    2. Advise him to wear knee-length stockings.
    3. Instruct him to soak both feet in cool water.
    4. Caution him not to exercise daily.

127. Correct answer - 1. Encourage the client to avoid caffeine and nicotine because they constrict vessels and would further impair his circulation; this includes encouraging the client to quit smoking or chewing tobacco, to avoid drinking caffeine-containing beverages, and not to ingest such drugs as amphetamines. Option 2 would impair circulation. Option 3: The client should keep the extremities warm and dry. Option 4: This client should exercise daily, unless he experiences pain.
CN: Physiological integrity

128. A 27-year-old-woman is admitted with complaints of severe fatigue, muscle weakness, and anorexia. She states she is recovering from the flu and has had severe nausea, frequent vomiting, and diarrhea. Blood is drawn for serum electrolyte measurements. Based on this client's symptoms, which finding should the nurse expect the laboratory report to show?
1. Below normal calcium level.
2. Below normal sodium level.
3. Below normal potassium level.
4. Above normal calcium level.

128. Correct answer - 3. Lack of potassium intake (related to anorexia and nausea) plus potassium loss by way of gastric secretions (from vomiting) and intestinal fluids (from diarrhea) puts this client at risk for a below-normal serum potassium level. Options 1 and 4 do not alter the body's calcium level; calcium is stored in bone and is not affected by GI changes. Option 2: Vomiting may increase the serum sodium level.
CN: Physiological integrity

129. Which intervention would best help to decrease ICP in a client with a head injury?
1. Placing client on hyperthermia blanket and elevating the body temperature above 99° F.
2. Elevating the HOB, increasing cerebral venous outflow.
3. Decreasing oxygen concentration to increase $PaCO_2$ level.
4. Place client in a supine position, increasing cerebral venous outflow.

129. Correct answer - 2. Elevating the HOB helps increase cerebral venous return and decrease ICP. Option 1: Elevating the body temperature also increases the metabolic rate and thereby increases the oxygen needs of the body. However, it does not decrease ICP. Option 3: Increasing the carbon dioxide levels in the blood causes vasodilation and thus increases ICP. Option 4: A supine position would decrease cerebral venous outflow and increase ICP.
CN: Physiological integrity

130. An 18-year-old male develops diabetes insipidus after a severe closed head injury. Which assessment findings would indicate that he also has hypernatremia?
1. Anorexia, muscle cramps, and a serum sodium level above 135 mEq/liter.
2. Numbness, muscle cramps, and a positive Trousseau's sign.
3. Cardiac arrhythmias, muscle weakness, nausea, and vomiting.
4. Thirst, dry and swollen tongue, and disorientation.

130. Correct answer 4. Diabetes insipidus results from lack of antidiuretic hormone, which causes significant urine losses. Such losses, in turn, lead to hypernatremia, which causes dry, sticky mucous membranes, thirst, swollen tongue, and disorientation. Option 1: A serum sodium level of 135 mEq/liter is within the normal range, and muscle cramps are a sign of hyponatremia. Option 2: Numbness and a positive Trousseau's sign indicate hypocalcemia. Option 3: Muscle irritability, not weakness, is characteristic of hypernatremia.
CN: Physiological integrity

131. A 52-year-old woman is admitted with a diagnosis of Cushing's syndrome. When analyzing her laboratory data, what would the nurse expect to find?
     1. Hyperglycemia, an increased white blood cell (WBC) count, and elevated cortisol and 17-ketosteroid levels.
     2. A decreased WBC count, hyponatremia, metabolic acidosis, and hyperglycemia.
     3. Glycosuria, hyperkalemia, a decreased cortisol level, and metabolic alkalosis.
     4. Decreased 17-ketosteroid levels, an elevated serum glucose level, hypocalcemia, and hyponatremia.

131. Correct answer - 1. In clients with Cushing's syndrome (hyperadrenalism), laboratory findings typically include sustained hyperglycemia, elevated cortisol and 17-ketosteroid levels, elevated WBC count, hypernatremia, hypokalemia, and metabolic alkalosis. Option 2: These would not be decreased in Cushing's syndrome. Options 3 and 4: Cushing's syndrome does not cause decreased cortisol level and hyperkalemia or hyponatremia and hypocalcemia.
     CN: Physiological integrity

HOW TO SCORE AND USE THE DIAGNOSTIC PROFILE

In the top "QUESTION NUMBER" row of boxes, mark each question number you answered wrong. Under each question number, check the box in the "TEST TAKING SKILLS" section that is the most appropriate reason you answered the question incorrectly. Do the same for the "CLIENT NEED CATEGORIES" section. The client need category code follows the rationale. Total the number of check marks, by line, in the "Totals" column. This provides you with a profile of your weak areas that should be improve upon prior to taking the NCLEX-RN.

PERSONAL DIAGNOSTIC PROFILE

QUESTION NUMBER																					Totals
TEST-TAKING SKILLS																					
Misread the question																					
Missed important point																					
Forgot fact or concept																					
Applied wrong fact or concept																					
Drew wrong conclusion																					
Incorrectly evaluated distractors																					
Mistakenly selected answer choice																					
Read into question																					
Made a wrong guess																					
Misunderstood question																					
CLIENT NEED CATEGORIES																					
Safe, effective care environment																					
Physiological integrity																					
Psychosocial integrity																					
Health promotion and maintenance																					

CALCULATION OF SUBSCORES

After you score your test, determine your subscores in these client need categories by filling in the following grid.

CLIENT NEED

	Safe, effective care environment	Physiological integrity	Psychosocial integrity	Health promotion & maintenance
Number of questions	39	81	2	9
Number incorrect				
Number correct				
Percent correct*				

*To determine the percent correct in each category, divide the number of items answered correctly by the total number of items and multiply the result by 100.

Note: This is a short test with a limited sample of items in each category. Therefore, if a score in any category is less than 75% correct, further study is strongly advised.

CHAPTER 6

Maternity Nursing Skill Test

TAKING THIS SKILL TEST

Your Study Guide Module has instructed you to take the following skill test after you have completed your review of the clinical area. This test will give you needed experience in answering NCLEX-RN type questions and will give you a good idea of your competence in this clinical area.

The format of the skill test gives you instant feedback as you take it. Each question is in the left column. The correct answer with rationale is in the right column. As you read the question in the left-hand column, cover the right-hand column with an index card until you have selected your answer. Slide the card down, keeping remaining question answers covered. When you have completed the test, use the Personal Diagnostic Profile to record why you answered any question incorrectly.

If you scored lower than 75% on this skill test, you should analyze the reason and go back and do further review. You may also wish to consult a current nursing textbook for any areas that are unclear to you.

1. A 30-year-old primigravida has just been told that she is 8 weeks pregnant. She tells the nurse, "My husband and I have been hoping to have a child for several years. Now I'm not so sure about having a baby." Which of these responses by the nurse would be *best?*
   1. "You've been wanting to become pregnant?"
   2. "Being pregnant will change your way of living?"
   3. "Most women at the beginning of pregnancy feel as you do."
   4. "You're having mixed feelings about the pregnancy."

2. A client who is 26 weeks pregnant has a routine check-up. Which laboratory test result should be called to her health care provider's attention?
   1. Urinary pH: 6.0
   2. White blood cells: 9,000/mm^3
   3. Hemoglobin: 10 g/dl
   4. Urinary specific gravity: 1.015

3. A 27-year-old client who is 12 weeks pregnant has had insulin-dependent diabetes since she was 15 years old. The nurse's teaching plan should include information related to the fact that pregnancy and diabetes will predispose her to which of these types of vaginitis?
   1. Trichomonas
   2. Monilial
   3. Hemophilus
   4. Desquamative inflammatory

1. Correct answer - 4. The client is expressing ambivalence, which is a normal response to pregnancy. The nurse acknowledges these mixed feelings in a matter-of-fact statement. Options 1 and 2: The nurse avoids the client's expressed feelings and changes the subject. Option 3: The nurse minimizes the client's feelings by focusing on "most women" rather than the client.
CN: Health promotion and maintenance

2. Correct answer - 3. A hemoglobin of 10 g/dl or less during pregnancy is indication of anemia. Option 2: The white blood cell count is within normal limits for the second trimester of pregnancy (normal range=5,000 to 15,000/mm^3). Options 1 and 4: The urine laboratory values are within normal limits.
CN: Health promotion and maintenance

3. Correct answer - 2. Monilial infections are commonly seen in women with diabetes because the organism (Candida albicans) thrives in a carbohydrate-rich milieu. Options 1, 3, and 4 are not more common in women with diabetes.
CN: Health promotion and maintenance

4. A pregnant client is scheduled to have an ultrasonogram to confirm the gestational age of the fetus. To prepare the client for the procedure, the nurse's instruction should include:
   1. "Take a mild laxative the evening prior to the procedure."
   2. "Take nothing by mouth for 8 hours prior to the procedure."
   3. "Drink at least 1 quart of water 2 hours prior to the procedure."
   4. "Empty your bladder immediately before the procedure."

4. Correct answer - 3. The woman is directed to come for the examination with a full bladder because it supports the uterus in position for the imaging. Options 1 and 2: There is no need to take a laxative or to remain NPO prior to the procedure. Option 4: If her bladder is empty, the test may be delayed for about 1 hour until she is able to fill it.
   CN: Safe, effective care environment

5. A 16-year-old primigravida has been receiving regular prenatal care. At 36 weeks gestation, she has symptoms of pregnancy-induced hypertension and is hospitalized. She is receiving I.V. magnesium sulfate therapy. The major goal of this therapy is to
   1. increase fetal lung maturity.
   2. increase the placental blood flow.
   3. decrease the possibility of premature labor.
   4. decrease the possibility of convulsions.

5. Correct answer - 4. Magnesium sulfate, an anticonvulsant and smooth muscle relaxant, is given to prevent convulsions. Option 1, 2, and 3: The drug has no effect on fetal lung maturity, placental blood flow, or premature labor.
   CN: Health promotion and maintenance

6. A 2-day-old newborn has the following laboratory results: hemoglobin, 18 g/dl; white blood cells, 25,000/mm^3; serum bilirubin, 7 mg/dl. Given these data, the nurse should obtain additional information by assessing which of these questions?
   1. Does the infant have an elevated temperature?
   2. Are the sclerae of the infant's eyes jaundiced?
   3. Does the infant have irregular respirations?
   4. Are the infant's hands and feet cyanotic?

6. Correct answer - 2. Physiologic jaundice, caused by increased breakdown of red blood cells and elevated serum bilirubin, is visible when the serum bilirubin level is above 5 mg/dl. The other laboratory data are within normal limits for the newborn. Option 1: There is no indication for checking temperature. Options 3 and 4: Irregular respirations and bluish discoloration of the hands and feet (acrocyanosis) are normally seen in the newborn.
   CN: Health promotion and maintenance

7. A client in the second stage of labor is observed to be holding her breath for 8 or 10 seconds at a time while pushing with each contraction. Based on this observation, the nurse should investigate which of these questions?
   1. Is she having carpopedal spasms?
   2. Is there evidence of crowning?
   3 What is the fetal heart rate?
   4. What is the client's blood pressure?

7. Correct answer - 3. Holding the breath for more than 5 seconds at a time can diminish the perfusion of oxygen across the placenta and result in fetal hypoxia, which would be manifested by a decrease in fetal heart rate. Option 1: Carpopedal spasms may occur with hyperventilation associated with pant-blow breathing during the earlier, transitional stage. Options 2 and 4: Fetal crowning and increased maternal blood pressure are expected during the second stage but are not related to breath-holding.
CN: Health promotion and maintenance

8. A client in early labor has an external fetal monitor applied to her abdomen. The monitor strip indicates occasional early decelerations of the fetal heart rate. Which of these actions should the nurse take?
   1. Continue with the client's plan of care.
   2. Reposition the transducer on the client's abdomen.
   3. Administer oxygen to the client.
   4. Elevate the client's legs while more information is obtained.

8. Correct answer - 1. Early deceleration (slowing of fetal heart rate) in response to compression of the fetal head is normal and usually does not indicate fetal distress. Option 2: There is no indication to reposition the transducer. Option 3: Oxygen would be administered in the case of severe variable decelerations. Option 4: The client's legs would be elevated if maternal hypotension were associated with late decelerations.
CN: Health promotion and maintenance

9. A client in labor is having contractions every 5 minutes, lasting 40 seconds. Her cervix is dilated 3 cm. The nurse should help her during contractions by reinforcing the technique of
   1. pant-blow breathing.
   2. abdominal breathing.
   3. slow, rhythmic chest breathing.
   4. shallow, light chest breathing.

9. Correct answer - 3. The client in early labor is encouraged to concentrate on slow, rhythmic chest breathing (six to nine breaths per minute) through the contraction. Option 1: Pant-blow breathing is used during the transitional phase. Options 2 and 4: When cervical dilatation reaches 5 cm, a change to shallower, lighter chest breathing, or abdominal breathing may be suggested.
CN: Health promotion and maintenance

10. A client is to get $Rh_0(D)$ immune globulin (RhoGAM). The nurse instructs her about the purpose and administration of RhoGAM. Which of these comments by the client indicates the need for *further* instruction?
    1. "I need RhoGAM because I have developed antibodies to my baby's Rh-positive blood."
    2. "If I ever have a miscarriage, I will need to be given RhoGAM again."
    3. "I must be given RhoGAM within 3 days of delivery for it to be effective."
    4. "I will be getting RhoGAM by an injection into a muscle."

10. Correct answer - 1. RhoGAM must be given *before* the mother produces antibodies to fetal cells that entered her bloodstream when the placenta separated. It has no effect if antibodies are already present in the maternal bloodstream. If the mother's indirect Coombs' test is negative and the infant's direct Coombs' test is negative, the mother is given RhoGAM within 72 hours of birth. Options 2, 3, and 4 are accurate and require no further instruction.
CN: Health promotion and maintenance

11. Which of these statements given by a postpartum client indicates a high risk for developing thrombophlebitis?
    1. "This was my eighth baby and the most difficult delivery of all."
    2. "I'm 29 years old and felt exhausted during this pregnancy."
    3. "I've needed to take medication for strong afterpains with this delivery."
    4. "This pregnancy was difficult because I was so constipated throughout it."

11. Correct answer - 1. Multiparity and a complicated delivery are associated with high risk for developing thrombophlebitis. Options 2, 3, and 4: Risk factors for thrombophlebitis do not include fatigue during pregnancy, afterpains, or constipation during pregnancy.
CN: Physiological integrity

12. A newborn female infant is transferred from the delivery room to the nursery. When the infant is 36 hours old, the nurse makes the following observations of her. Which finding should be investigated further?
    1. Fine, downy hair over forehead and ears.
    2. Positive Babinski's sign.
    3. Abduction of hips to 45 degrees.
    4. Mucoid vaginal discharge.

12. Correct answer - 3. Hips normally abduct to more than 60 degrees. Abduction to 45 degrees suggests developmental hip dysplasia. Options 1, 2, and 4: These other findings are normal findings in the newborn.
CN: Health promotion and maintenance

13. A newborn, infected with the HIV virus, has been assessed as small for gestational age and defined facial characteristics. What are the facial characteristics seen in a newborn with HIV?
    1. Microcephalic, epicanthal folds, and flattened philtrum.
    2. Flat nasal bridge, slanted eyes and protruding tongue.
    3. Microcephalic, prominent, boxlike forehead and patulous lips.
    4. Hydrocephalic, bulging fontanels and "setting sun eyes."

13. Correct answer - 3. HIV-infected infants have characteristic facies of microcephaly, prominent boxlike forehead, patulous lips, flattened nasal bridge and distancing of the canthus. Option 1: This is the facies of fetal alcohol syndrome. Option 2: This is the facies of Trisomy 21. Option 4: This is the facies of hydrocephalus.
    CN: Physiological integrity

14. At 1 minute and 5 minutes after birth, the nurse assesses an infant that has an apical heart rate of 104 and 110, flexed, crying, and cyanotic to acrocyanotic. What action should the nurse take next?
    1. Initiate CPR.
    2. Let the mother hold the infant.
    3. Apply identification bracelets.
    4. Maintain a patent airway.

14. Correct answer - 4. This infant's APGAR score is 8 at 1 minute and 9 at 5 minutes. The nurse's priority is to maintain a patent airway. Option 1: CPR is not indicated for this infant. Option 2: Bonding is important, but a patent airway and drying the infant are priorities. Option 3: Identification bracelets need to be completed as part of the delivery process but are not the immediate priority.
    CN: Safe, effective care environment

15. A client in her second trimester of pregnancy calls the clinic complaining of light, white, vaginal discharge. She denies itching, foul-odor or a temperature. What are the home instructions for this client?
    1. Do a vinegar douche daily for the next 2 days and call the clinic in 3 days.
    2. Continue daily bathing, and wear cotton underwear; call if discharge increases.
    3. Use over-the-counter Monistat cream as directed and call if discharge worsens.
    4. Wear a tampon until discharge decreases.

15. Correct answer - 2. This client is describing a normal discharge of leukorrhea that occurs in pregnancy. Daily bathing and cotton underwear should minimize this problem. Option 1: Douching is contraindicated for pregnant women. Option 3: A pregnant client is at a higher risk for developing a Candida infection, but these symptoms are not what this client has described. Option 4: Pregnant women should not wear tampons at any time.
    CN: Physiological integrity

16. A client in labor is crying, having contractions every 2 or 3 minutes, lasting 60 seconds. Her cervix is dilated to 6 cm, 80% effaced, and there is a small amount of discharge from the vagina. What phase of labor is this client in?
    1. Active   3. Transition
    2. Latent   4. Descent

16. Correct answer - 1. The cervix is dilated to 6 cm and 80% effaced, indicating active phase, stage 1 labor. Option 2: The client is further progressed in the labor process. Option 3: The client is not dilated to 8 cm yet. Option 4: This is a phase of second-stage labor.
    CN: Physiological integrity

17. A client that is at 36 weeks gestation has just been involved in an automobile accident as a driver of the car. The client says she was wearing her seat belt. This client is at an increased risk for developing which high-risk prenatal condition?
    1. Placenta previa
    2. Incompetent cervix
    3. Pregnancy induced hypertension
    4. Abruptio placenta

17. Correct answer - 4. Blunt trauma to the abdomen is one cause of abruptio placenta. Abruptio placenta is a premature separation from the uterine wall. Option 1: Placenta previa is implantation in the lower segment of the uterine well. An automobile accident does not cause this. Option 2: Incompetent cervix occurs in the 4th or 5th month of pregnancy. Option 3: PIH is indicated by hypertension, edema and proteinuria. An automobile accident does not cause this.
CN: Physiological integrity

18. A client has just had a fetal monitoring test in which there were two instances of fetal heart rate acceleration of 15 bpm, lasting 15 seconds in a 10-minute time frame. What type of fetal monitoring test was done?
    1. A reactive non-stress test
    2. A non-reactive non-stress test
    3. A positive non-stress test
    4. A negative non-stress test

18. Correct answer - 1. A reactive NST shows at least two 15 bpm accelerations of FHR lasting 15 seconds or more with fetal movement over 20 minutes. There is institutional variation.
CN: Physiological integrity

19. The nurse is teaching breast-feeding to a new mother. Which hormone stimulates the alveolar cells of the breast to promote milk production?
    1. Estrogen
    2. Progesterone
    3. Prolactin
    4. Oxytocin

19. Correct answer - 3. Prolactin is secreted by the anterior pituitary to promote milk production. Option 1: Estrogen levels drop after delivery. Option 2: Progesterone levels drop after delivery. Option 4: Oxytocin levels are increased with breast-feeding sucking. They affect the contractility of the myometrium.
CN: Physiological integrity

20. The client is planning to continue breast-feeding her baby after she returns work. She asks the nurse if she can express and store milk. How long can breast milk be stored?
    1. 8 hours at room temperature.
    2. 14 days in the refrigerator.
    3. 14 days in the freezer unit of the refrigerator.
    4. 8 months in the freezer unit of the refrigerator.

20. Correct answer - 3. Breast milk can be stored in the freezer unit of a refrigerator for 2 weeks. It can be stored in glass or plastic containers. It should be thawed by running warm water over the container, never microwaving it. Option 1: 6 hours at room temperature is the longest recommended time. Option 2: Up to 5 days storage in the refrigerator is recommended. Option 4: Only 2 weeks storage in a freezer unit of the refrigerator, up to 6 months in a separate freezer unit.
CN: Health promotion and maintenance

21. A client of 20 weeks gestation arrives for her prenatal visit on a cold winter day in January. The physician, reviewing her history, recommends an immunization. Which immunization would most likely be recommended?
    1. MMR (measles, mumps, rubella)
    2 Influenza
    3. Poliomyelitis
    4. Rhotashield

22. A newborn male born into a Jewish family will be circumcised after discharge from the hospital. How will this be reflected in the discharge teaching plan?
    1. It will not be included in the plan because this is not a current infant problem.
    2. The family will be asked if they are familiar with circumcision care.
    3. A brochure on circumcision will be included with the discharge papers.
    4. The parents' cultural base will be assessed and a plan of circumcision care developed.

23. A 26-week pregnant client is having back pain. Which of the following comfort measures should the nurse teach her?
    1. Perform pelvic rocking exercises.
    2. Apply moist heat to her lower back.
    3. Take frequent rest periods.
    4. Have her husband rub her back.

21. Correct answer - 2. Influenza vaccine is recommended for women greater than 14 weeks gestation during influenza season. Options 1 and 3 are live viruses and are contraindicated in pregnancy. Option 4: Rotashield is for rotavirus and given to children under the age of 2 years.
CN: Health promotion and maintenance

22. Correct answer - 4. A family cultural assessment is a part of the newborn's history. The discharge teaching should define circumcision care and provide anticipatory guidance. Option 1: This is a planned procedure for this infant and needs to be addressed. Option 2: This could be a beginning base of questioning, but needs to be further facilitated. Option 3: A brochure with no verbal explanation should never be given alone as part of the discharge teaching plan.
CN: Health promotion and maintenance

23. Correct answer - 1. Pelvic rocking exercises relieve back strain and strengthen the abdominal muscles, providing for sustained relief. Option 2: Moist heat is not an appropriate treatment for a nurse to prescribe in this situation. Option 3: Frequent rest periods are important but not as effective as pelvic rocking. Option 4: Back rubs may provide temporary, but not sustained, relief.
CN: Physiological integrity

24. A woman with gestational diabetes delivers a 6-lb 2-oz girl at 36 weeks. The newborn is now in the NICU with respiratory distress. Which is the *most* therapeutic statement to make to the mother, who is extremely upset?
    1. "Your baby will be fine because her weight is appropriate for your length of pregnancy."
    2. "I know how difficult this must be for you. I had an aunt whose baby died when she delivered early."
    3. "You may be feeling helpless and overwhelmed now with what you may not have expected."
    4. "I'm sure you are glad to have labor over since you had such a difficult pregnancy."

24. Correct answer - 3. This addresses the feelings the client is probably experiencing, lets her verbalize more freely, and conveys acceptance of her feelings. Option 1 gives false reassurance. Option 2 is inappropriate. Option 4 is nonsupportive and does not deal with her feelings.
CN: Physiological integrity

25. You are responsible for giving the initial feeding of sterile water to a newborn. The mother asks why you are feeding her baby sterile water. What is your *best* response?
    1. "Sterile water is less harmful, if he aspirates some."
    2. "The doctor always orders this."
    3. "Glucose water would give the baby too many calories."
    4. "Formula should be withheld for 12 hours."

25. Correct answer - 1. Plain sterile water is less irritating to the respiratory tract if any is aspirated. Sterile water is best for the initial feeding. Option 2 is untrue. Options 3 and 4: Glucose water and formula if aspirated can cause an inflammatory response and pneumonia.
CN: Physiological integrity

26. What intervention would *best* keep a client's nipples in good condition for breast-feeding and to prevent infection?
    1. Wash the nipples with soap and water before each feeding.
    2. Expose the nipples to air and sunlight for short periods.
    3. Use a plastic bra liner to handle leakage.
    4. Cleanse the nipples with a mild antiseptic solution.

26. Correct answer - 2. Exposing the nipples to air and sunlight will help toughen them. Option: 1 and 4: Soap and antiseptics should not be used on the nipples because they remove protective oils that keep nipples supple. Option 3: Plastic bra liners are not recommended because they retain moisture against the nipples.
CN: Health promotion and maintenance

27. When caring for a newborn receiving phototherapy, the nurse should
    1. decrease the amount of the infant's formula.
    2. dress the infant warmly.
    3. massage the infant's skin with lotion.
    4. give the infant fluids every 3 hours.

27. Correct answer - 4. Phototherapy causes insensible water loss. Fluids should be provided to avoid dehydration. Option 1: Fluid intake should be increased. Formula is mostly liquid and would aid in reducing risk of dehydration. Option 2: The infant is undressed in order to expose as much skin surface as possible. The eyes are covered to protect them from the light. An abbreviated diaper may be worn. Option 3: The infant's skin should be clean and patted dry. No lotion is used on the skin surfaces to interfere with the phototherapy.
    CN: Physiological integrity

28. A pregnant client has a stress test done at 36 weeks gestation. Which result indicates an adequate oxygen reserve?
    1. Positive
    2. Negative
    3. Reactive
    4. Nonreactive

28. Correct answer - 2. A negative stress test indicates the fetus is experiencing an adequate oxygen reserve. Option 1 would indicate the need for further testing. Options 3 and 4 are related to the results of a non-stress test.
    CN: Health promotion and maintenance

29. A client is breast-feeding her baby for the first time. How long should she be taught to allow the infant to nurse on each breast?
    1. 5 to 7 minutes.
    2. 10 to 15 minutes.
    3. 20 minutes.
    4. As long as the infant will suck.

29. Correct answer - 4. Feeding time should be on infant demand. Usually the infant will feed 10 or 15 minutes on first breast and as long as necessary on second breast. Options 1, 2, and 3: Time limits should not be placed on the infant.
    CN: Health promotion and maintenance

30. A 38-year-old gravida 1 para 0 has been progressing normally during her first 36 weeks. At 37 weeks gestation, she comes to her prenatal appointment with complaints of headaches and difficulty seeing. In assessing the client, the nurse should expect to find
    1. uterine tenderness and temperature of 101° F.
    2. glucosuria and pulse rate of 100 bpm.
    3. respirations of 24 per minute and productive cough.
    4. blood pressure of 160/106 mm Hg and pitting ankle edema

30. Correct answer - 4. The symptoms suggest the client may have pregnancy-induced hypertension, which could lead to preeclampsia. Therefore, the nurse should expect the client to have an elevated blood pressure and peripheral edema. Options 1, 2 and 3 are not consistent with the symptoms.
    CN: Physiological integrity

31. A woman who delivered a healthy boy 12 hours ago plans to breast-feed. When the nurse brings the baby, who is awake and alert, to the mother's room, she is asleep. Which action should the nurse take?
    1. Give the infant a clear liquid feeding.
    2. Return the infant to the nursery until the mother awakes.
    3. Wake the mother and encourage her to feed her baby.
    4. Report this situation to the nurse manager.

31. Correct answer - 3. Mothers who are breast-feeding should be encouraged to nap between feedings. Infants who are breast-feeding should be fed when they are awake and alert. When breast feeding first begins, the infant should be put to breast so it adapts to breast-feeding and obtains colostrum, containing antibodies. The infant at the breast stimulates the production of breast milk. Options 1, 2, and 4: These actions would not advance the breast-feeding process.
    CN: Health promotion and maintenance

32. A primigravida client who is 8 weeks pregnant attends the antepartal clinic for the first time. She should be taught to contact the clinic, immediately, if she develops which of these symptoms?
    1. Persistent headache
    2. Difficulty in sleeping
    3. Recurrent heartburn
    4. Urinary frequency

32. Correct answer - 1. Persistent headache is a danger sign in pregnancy, as it may indicate hypertension. Option 2: Difficulty in sleeping is not a danger sign in pregnancy. Options 3 and 4 are normal in pregnant women.
    CN: Health promotion and maintenance

33. A woman who is 16 weeks pregnant has an amniocentesis. Which instruction should be given to her after the procedure is completed?
    1. "Stay in bed for at least 8 hours."
    2. "Wear a sanitary pad to absorb the vaginal drainage."
    3. "Notify your health care provider if you have any contractions."
    4. "Increase your fluid intake for the next 24 hours."

33. Correct answer - 3. Following amniocentesis, the woman should be instructed to report the onset of uterine contractions, abdominal pain, vaginal discharge, chills, and fetal hyperactivity or lack of activity. Option 1: Bedrest for 8 hours is not necessary following this procedure. Option 2: There should be no vaginal discharge. Option 4: It is not necessary to increase fluid intake to replace the small amount of fluid removed during amniocentesis.
    CN: Physiological integrity

34. A primigravida is admitted to the hospital in labor. Her cervix is fully dilated. She asks the nurse for some medication for pain. The nurse's response should be based on which understanding about the effects of pain medication given at this time?
    1. It may interfere with her ability to bond with her baby.
    2. It may lower her blood pressure to a hazardous level.
    3. It may cause a precipitous delivery.
    4. It may affect the baby's adaptation to extrauterine life.

34. Correct answer - 4. Administering analgesia during the second stage of labor may affect the fetus and result in difficulty following birth. Option 1: Bonding during the postpartum period should not be affected by analgesia given during labor. Option 2: During normal labor, analgesia would not lower blood pressure to a hazardous level. Option 3: Analgesia is more likely to delay delivery than to cause precipitous delivery.
    CN: Physiological integrity

35. A 23-year-old primigravida is admitted to the labor unit at 40 weeks gestation. After several hours, her labor has not progressed. An oxytocin infusion is prescribed. Forty-five minutes after it is started, uterine contractions occur every $1^1/_2$ minutes, with incomplete uterine relaxation between contractions. Which action should the nurse take?
    1. Stop the infusion, keep the line open and turn her on her left side.
    2. Maintain the infusion and monitor fetal heart rate.
    3. Slow the infusion, keep the line open and make her comfortable.
    4. Maintain the infusion and have her pant and blow with contractions.

35. Correct answer - 1. Prolonged contractions with incomplete uterine relaxation between contractions necessitates discontinuing the infusion and positioning client on left side for optimal maternal fetal circulation to prevent severe fetal hypoxia and rupture of the uterus. Option 2: The infusion should be discontinued. Continuing the infusion will increase the risks. Option 3: The infusion should be discontinued. Option 4: The infusion should be discontinued; panting and blowing will not reduce the danger of the situation.
CN: Physiological integrity

36. A baby boy who is breast-feeding refuses to eat on the second day of his birth. His mother begins to cry and says, "Nothing is going right. He won't eat and I still haven't been able to have a bowel movement." Which phase of postpartum restoration is she most likely experiencing?
    1. Taking-in
    2. Taking-hold
    3. Postpartal blues
    4. Let-down

36. Correct answer - 2. During the taking-hold phase (days 2-3), the mother is interested in resuming control of her bodily functions and is concerned about her ability to successfully mother her child. Option 1: The taking-in phase is the first period of postpartum restoration and is characterized by maternal passivity and dependency. Preoccupation with her own needs, rather than those of the infant, is usual. Options 3 and 4: Postpartum blues is a transient period of depression manifested by tearing, anorexia and difficulty sleeping. A "let-down" feeling may accompany postpartum blues. However, this client's symptoms are not typical of postpartum blues.
CN: Health promotion and maintenance

37. A breast-feeding mother reports that her baby spits up after each feeding. What is the best action for the nurse to take?
    1. Demonstrate the proper technique for burping the infant.
    2. Return the infant to the nursery for close observation.
    3. Feed the infant sterile water and allow the mother to watch.
    4. Observe the mother and infant during the next feeding period.

37. Correct answer - 4. Many neonates regurgitate following a feeding. Observing the mother and infant at the next feeding will let the nurse assess the situation and determine if there is a feeding problem. Option 1: A decision to teach burping technique would be made only after it is determined that the mother's technique is incorrect or that she needs instruction. Options 2 and 3 are not the initial nursing actions indicated, although they could be indicated later if the infant has definite feeding problems.
CN: Health promotion and maintenance

38. A client has been diagnosed as having early pregnancy-induced hypertension. Which of the following dietary instructions should the nurse include for this client?
    1. Force fluids
    2. High protein
    3. Eliminate sodium
    4. Low carbohydrates

38. Correct answer - 2. The recommended diet should be high in protein to replace the protein loss in the urine. Options 1 and 3: Sodium and fluid intake are usually regulated. Sodium should not be eliminated and fluids are not forced. Option 4: Carbohydrate intake should not be reduced.
    CN: Physiological integrity

39. A 17-year-old client is 28 weeks pregnant with her first child and has been followed regularly at the antepartal clinic. The last 2 weeks, she has gained 6 pounds. What is the *best* interpretation of a weight gain of 6 pounds in 2 weeks in a client who is in the 28th week of pregnancy?
    1. It indicates a poor understanding of good nutritional practices.
    2. It indicates a health problem in a teenage primigravida.
    3. It is due to causes other than an excessive caloric intake.
    4. It is expected for this period of gestation.

39. Correct answer - 3. Weight gain may be from fluid retention and pregnancy-induced hypertension. Option 1: Weight gain may be unrelated to good nutritional practices. Option 2: Weight gain may or may not be indicative of a problem. Option 4: A weight gain of 6 pounds in 2 weeks during the third trimester is greater than expected.
    CN: Health promotion and maintenance

40. A client refuses to get out of bed on the 2nd postpartum day, even though she was to be up 8 hours after delivery. When asked why, she states, "I bleed so much more when I stand up." What is the *best* action for the nurse to take?
    1. Have the client sit on the side of the bed and dangle her feet.
    2. Explain the relationship between gravity, activity and increased lochial flow.
    3. Explain that postpartum bleeding is not really bleeding, but a kind of menstrual flow.
    4. Ask her if other women in her family had a similar experience after delivery.

40. Correct answer - 2. The recumbent position causes pooling of lochia in the vagina and uterus and this accumulation is discharged when the client stands. Options 1 and 4 are not indicated because they do not respond to the client's immediate concerns and are not relevant to the situation. Option 3: Lochia is similar to the menstrual flow in that it is nonoffensive. However, its purpose is to rid the uterus of debris remaining after delivery and its composition is different from that of the menstrual flow.
    CN: Health promotion and maintenance

41. To provide safe care for a client during the induction of labor, the nurse should monitor which data during the Pitocin administration?
    1. Amniotic fluid status
    2. Cervical dilation
    3. Urine output
    4. Contraction characteristics

41. Correct answer - 4. Pitocin is a potent stimulant of the myometrium. Contractions that are strong, occurring less than every 2 minutes, and lasting 60 seconds or more interfere with the oxygen supply to the uterus and the fetus. Options 1, 2, and 3: Although amniotic fluid status, urinary output, and cervical dilation are important, the most important assessment during Pitocin administration is monitoring uterine contractions (duration, strength, frequency).
    CN: Physiological integrity

42. While performing a vaginal examination on a client in labor, the nurse feels the umbilical cord. Which action should the nurse take *first?*
    1. Relieve pressure on the cord.
    2. Gently replace the cord.
    3. Note the tension of the cord.
    4. Apply a moist sponge to the cord.

42. Correct answer - 1. When an umbilical cord prolapse is identified, pressure on the cord by the presenting part must be relieved. This will help restore fetal circulation and supply oxygen to the fetus. Options 2 and 3 would cause additional trauma to the umbilical cord. Option 4: If the umbilical cord is exposed, placing a moist sponge is important; however, it is secondary to relieving the pressure.
    CN: Physiological integrity

43. To promote comfort for a client who is in early labor, which of the following should be included on her care plan?
    1. Encourage pelvic rocking exercises.
    2. Encourage rapid breathing patterns.
    3. Encourage sacral massage.
    4. Encourage walking with assistance.

43. Correct answer - 4. In early labor, many women are more comfortable when walking. Options 1 and 3 are more appropriate measures in the active phase if back pain is present. Option 2: Accelerated breathing patterns are used as a coping method when labor becomes more intense.
    CN: Physiological integrity

44. A client is very concerned about taking her newborn home. Her husband is a second-grade teacher and a child in his class had been sent home with chicken pox. Both parents had chickenpox in early childhood. What discharge teaching needs to be given to this mother?
    1. "It is best if you go home and the baby remains in isolation in the nursery."
    2. "Call us and let us know if your husband shows any signs of developing chicken pox."
    3. "The baby should not develop chicken pox because it is too young for this disease of later childhood."
    4. "The baby should not develop chicken pox because of passive immunity of IgG, and you already have antibodies to chicken pox."

44. Correct answer - 4. Maternally transported transplacentally IgG protects the newborn against bacterial and viral infections for which the mother already has antibodies. Option 1: The baby will have passive antibodies. An infected infant would be transferred out of newborn nursery. Option 2: The husband has immunity to chicken pox. If he did not have them he would have to wait the 14- to 21-day incubation period. Option 3: The baby has passive antibodies from the mother.
CN: Health promotion and maintenance

45. A 27-year-old primigravida has insulin-dependant diabetes. At 38 weeks gestation, she delivers a healthy 9-pound 9-ounce (4,320 g) baby girl and she plans to breast-feed her. The nurse should teach that breast-feeding
    1. should not be done by anyone with diabetes.
    2. will have no effect on her diabetes.
    3. by mothers with diabetes will require insulin adjustment.
    4. is discouraged because it will cause rapid blood glucose changes in the mother.

45. Correct answer - 3. An adjustment in diet and therefore in insulin requirements is necessary for the woman with diabetes mellitus who breast-feeds. Option 1: Breast-feeding is not necessarily contraindicated for women with diabetes. Option 2: Breast-feeding will have an effect on the mother's dietary and insulin requirements. Option 4: With appropriate dietary and insulin regulation, there should be no rapid blood glucose fluctuations in the diabetic mother.
CN: Health promotion and maintenance

46. A 28-year-old female is being seen in the emergency department for nausea, vomiting, and abdominal cramping. After initial exam and lab test results, it is determined the client is pregnant and using heroin. The client agrees to do anything you ask, she just wants help. What is the *best* treatment goal for this client's chemical dependency?
    1. Let her continue heroin use until she delivers.
    2. Discontinue all drug use immediately.
    3. Maintain her on methadone until she delivers.
    4. Discharge her from the emergency department with a phone number for the chemical dependency clinic.

46. Correct answer - 3. Heroin is a narcotic opioid. A heroin client is treated with methadone maintenance until delivery. Methadone blocks withdrawal symptoms, is in liquid form, and can be individualized to the lowest therapeutic level. Option 1: Continuing heroin use continues the pattern of high-risk outcomes for the mother and fetus. Option 2: Discontinuing use immediately may result in a stillborn birth. Option 4: A substance-abusing client needs immediate intervention, particularly when she is pregnant. This client will probably not follow-up with a phone number.
CN: Safe, effective care environment

47. Your pregnant client in labor has just asked you to assist her to an effective birthing position to shorten her second stage of labor. Which position would be best to accomplish that?
    1. Side-lying
    2. Squatting
    3. Lithotomy
    4. Hand-and-knees

47. Correct answer - 2. Squatting position increases the diameter of the pelvic outlet. There is a decrease in the amount of time spent in second stage and decreased lacerations and episiotomies. Option 1: Side-lying may be a more comfortable position but does not decrease second stage. Option 3: This position is frequently used in Western practices for convenience but doesn't decrease second stage of labor. Option 4: This position is helpful for non-reassuring fetal monitoring patterns.
CN: Safe, effective care environment

48. A 24 year old primigravida was being treated for pregnancy induced hypertension (PIH). Her condition progressed to the eclamptic state and a C-section has just been completed. She is being transferred to the ICU for hemolysis, elevated liver enzymes, and low platelets (HELLP) syndrome. What are the characteristics of HELLP syndrome?
    1. A condition of hemolysis, elevated liver enzymes, and low platelets.
    2. A condition of hypertension, extra liver load, and proteinuria
    3. A condition of hypertension, elevated liver, and low plasma.
    4. A condition in which medical help is frequently solicited.

48. Correct answer - 1. This condition indicates hepatic involvement and is evidenced by hemolysis, elevated liver enzymes, and low platelets. Option 2: These are not HELLP syndrome signs. Option 3: Hypertension may still occur, but the hemolysis and low platelets are the biggest problems at this time. Option 4: This is not why this is called HELLP syndrome.
CN: Physiological integrity

49. A 16-year-old primipara delivered 10 hours ago. She has called you to her bedside because she has saturated two pads in 1 hour. What action should you take *initially?*
    1. Leave the bedside and phone her health care provider.
    2. Get a set of vital signs.
    3. Open an I.V. that has 1,000 ml of D5L/R with 10 units of Pitocin added.
    4. Assess her fundus.

49. Correct answer - 4. The immediate intervention is to evaluate her uterus to determine if it is firmly contracted. Option 1: You would not leave the bedside until you have done further assessment and intervention for this client. You may need to phone her health care provider, but not first. Option 2: You will need a set of vital signs, but you must first determine uterine contractility. Option 3: You may increase her I.V. fluids after determining her uterine status. You will need a health care provider's order to increase rate and amount of Pitocin.
CN: Safe, effective care environment

50. A pregnant African-American client is a carrier for sickle cell trait. Her husband is also a carrier of the trait. What is their chance of bearing a child who will have sickle cell disease?
    1. There is no chance for them to have a child with sickle cell disease.
    2. All the children they bear will have sickle cell disease.
    3. All the children they bear will be carriers of sickle cell trait.
    4. There is a 25% chance they will bear a child with sickle cell disease.

50. Correct answer - 4. There is a one in four chance with each pregnancy they could produce a child with sickle cell disease. Sickle cell disease is an autosomal recessive disorder. Option 1: With each pregnancy, there is a one in four chance of producing a child with sickle cell disease. Option 2: With each pregnancy, there is a three in four chance of producing a child that will not have sickle cell disease. Option 3: With each pregnancy, there is a 50% chance that the child they bear will be a carrier of sickle cell trait.
CN: Health promotion and maintenance

51. An intrapartal client has just been given an epidural anesthesia to provide comfort during the labor process. Which of the following is an ominous sign, if occurring immediately after the epidural?
    1. Hypertension
    2. Euglycemia
    3. 2+ deep tendon reflexes
    4. Hypotension

51. Correct answer - 4. Hypotension is an indicator of a problem after epidural anesthesia, and warrants immediate attention. Option 1: Hypertension following an epidural anesthetic is transitory and occurs only if the client is anxious about the procedure. Option 2: This is normal glucose and not effected by the epidural anesthesia. Option 3: These are normal deep tendon reflexes.
CN: Safe, effective care environment

52. At a prenatal visit, a 28-week gestation client complains of sharp pain she gets occasionally in her lower abdomen and groin. She reports that it feels like it just "catches on something." Your *best* explanation should be that this is due to
    1. intensified Braxton-Hicks contractions.
    2. stretching of the pelvic ligaments.
    3. dilation of the ureters.
    4. a developing urinary tract infection.

52. Correct answer - 2. The "catching sensation" clients describe is the stretching of pelvic ligaments to compensate for the growth of the pregnant uterus. Option 1: The sensation she is describing is not Braxton-Hicks contractions, which would be a tightening and relaxation. Option 3: Dilation of the ureters does occur during pregnancy, but is usually unnoticed by the client. Option 4: The sensation she is describing is not indicative of a urinary tract infection.
CN: Physiological integrity

53. A client with systemic lupus erythematosus (SLE) comes to the clinic with an unplanned pregnancy. She thought she could not get pregnant with her disease. She asks what risk factors her disease will cause in pregnancy. What is the *best* explanation to give?
    1. "Now that you are pregnant, your disease will not be a risk factor."
    2. "You will need to increase your amount of anticonvulsants during pregnancy."
    3. " You will need to be observed more closely for kidney problems during pregnancy."
    4. "You will not be able to maintain this pregnancy because of your pre-existing condition."

53. Correct answer - 3. Because lupus is an autoimmune collagen disease, there is an increased workload on the kidneys. Option 1: This disease **is** a problem in pregnancy. Option 2: Anticonvulsants are used for the treatment of epilepsy. Option 4: The client will have a high-risk pregnancy. She is at increased risk of spontaneous abortion, stillbirth, prematurity, and SGA.
CN: Physiological integrity

54. A client who is gravida 3 para 0 has just been informed that she will need a Shirodkar-Barter procedure at 14 weeks gestation. She is crying and upset because she does not understand this procedure. What is the most accurate description of a Shirodkar-Barter procedure?
    1. "It provides implantation of the placenta in the correct location."
    2. "It repairs leaking of amniotic fluid."
    3. "It provides reinforcement for the cervix."
    4. "It allows for adequate pelvic stretching for delivery."

54. Correct answer - 3. The Shirodkar-Barter provides a tightening to reinforce a weak cervix. Option 1: This procedure does not alter implantation of the placenta. Option 2: This procedure does not repair leaking of amniotic fluid and would not be done if amniotic fluid was leaking. Option 4: This procedure does not effect pelvic stretching.
CN: Physiological integrity

55. A client has been in labor for 16 hours. She is now dilated to 9.6. She is crying and thrashing and yells, "I have to push now and get this baby out." What action should the nurse take?
    1. Call her health care provider to get pain medications to calm her.
    2. Tell her to "go ahead and push and see what happens."
    3. Catheterize her for residual urine.
    4. Help her regain control and coach her to pant.

55. Correct answer - 4. This client needs to get into control and save her energy for delivery. She needs direct coaching to pant so her cervix can finish dilatation to 10. She can then push for delivery. Option 1: This client can not have pain medications in the transition period. Option 2: If this client pushes, she will cause edema of the cervix, and prolong labor. Option 3: The client needs to get back under control. However, she may need to be catheterized, if she has not voided in 2 hours and a full bladder is impeding labor progress.
CN: Physiological integrity

56. Immediately after birth a newborn was dried, a hat was put on, and he was wrapped in a warm blanket and placed in his mother's arms. Using a warmed blanket prevents what mechanism of heat loss?
    1. Conduction
    2. Convection
    3. Evaporation
    4. Radiation

57. An woman with insulin-dependent diabetes is 32 weeks pregnant. She asks the nurse about her insulin needs for the remainder of her pregnancy. Which response, by the nurse, is *most* accurate? "Insulin needs will
    1. "increase as the placental hormones destroy insulin."
    2. "decrease as long as you do not develop an infection."
    3. "decrease as your pancreas will provide more insulin."
    4. "increase as the baby develops and puts on weight."

58. Assessment of a 12-hour-old infant reveals jaundice evident in the sclera and buccal mucosa. This requires further assessment for indications of
    1. normal physiological jaundice of the newborn.
    2. liver disease.
    3. a staphylococcal infection.
    4. anemia.

59. You are completing a newborn assessment. When you elicit the Moro reflex, the newborn responds asymmetrically. What should you do next?
    1. Ring a bell to see if the newborn responds to sound.
    2. Assess gluteal skin folds, looking for congenital hip disease.
    3. Palpate the clavicles for crepitus.
    4. Suction the newborn so you can again elicit the Moro reflex.

56. Correct answer - 1. Having a warmed blanket reduces the risk of heat loss from placing the infant near a colder object. Option 2: Convection is prevented by elimination of cool air currents. Option 3: Evaporation was prevented by drying the baby immediately after birth. Option 4: Radiation occurs when heat loss goes to a cool object, not in direct contact. CN: Safe, effective care environment

57. Correct answer - 1. A pregnant woman's insulin needs fluctuate throughout pregnancy. It is most likely that there will be a need for more insulin because of the production of the placental hormones, which are destructive to insulin. Options 2 and 3 are inaccurate statements. Option 4: Good prenatal care provides close surveillance for regulation of insulin needs; however, fetal development and weight gain will not increase insulin needs. CN: Physiological integrity

58. Correct answer - 2. Jaundice in the newborn prior to 24 hours of ages indicates liver disease, sepsis, blood incompatibilities, or maternal drug use. Option 1: Physiological jaundice occurs in more than 50% of newborns on days 3 to 5 of life, not in 12 hours. Option 3: Jaundice is not an indicator in a baby with a staphylococcal infection. Pustules are usually an indicator in this condition. Option 4: Anemia is indicated by pallor of the skin, not jaundice. CN: Physiological integrity

59. Correct answer - 3. Asymmetrical response of Moro is indicative of fracture of the clavicle, injury to the brachial plexus, or severe CNS damage. Option 1: Hearing deficit is not indicative of an asymmetrical Moro reflex. Option 2: Congenital hip disorder is not indicative of an asymmetrical Moro reflex. Option 4: Suctioning of the newborn makes no difference in eliciting a Moro reflex. CN: Physiological integrity

60. A full-term newborn, delivered by C-section 2 hours earlier, has a respiratory rate of 65, mild nasal flaring, and mild substernal retractions. His parents are requesting to begin breast-feeding. What action should the nurse take next?
    1. Take him to his mother's room and assist with breast-feeding teaching.
    2. Place the infant under a radiant warmer and assess his respiratory status.
    3. Leave the infant in the open crib by the desk and phone the health care provider.
    4. Suction the infant and reposition him on his right side.

60. Correct answer - 2. This infant is demonstrating respiratory distress, probably because of transient tachypnea. An infant with respiratory distress will increase its respiratory rate, have nasal flaring, retractions, grunting, and cyanosis. Further respiratory assessment needs to be done in a neutral thermal environment. Option 1: The infant's immediate need is adequate oxygenation, not nutrition. Option 3: The infant should be in a neutral thermal environment, and further evaluated before you phone the health care provider. Option 4: Suctioning this infant will not correct the problem of transient tachypnea.
CN: Physiological integrity

61. A client in preterm labor has just had a rupture of membranes. The amniotic fluid is light yellow and foul smelling. She vaginally delivers a 4-pound 5-ounce infant of 36 weeks gestation. The infant is transferred to the newborn nursery. What should the nursery nurse do *first?*
    1. Obtain blood, nasal, and ear cultures as ordered by the health care provider.
    2. Initiate Ampicillin and Gentamicin antibiotic treatment as ordered.
    3. Assess the infant's vital signs.
    4. Put on gloves prior to handling the infant.

61. Correct answer - 4. Put on clean gloves prior to handling any infant just delivered and brought to the nursery. This is part of universal precautions. Option 1: Cultures will need to be obtained, to rule out sepsis. This is *not* the first priority. Option 2: Antibiotic therapy will usually begin after cultures are obtained. This is *not* the first action. Option 3: This infant will need baseline vital signs. The nurse needs gloves on before handling this infant to get these.
CN: Safe, effective care environment

62. A client in early labor is using non-pharmacologic pain management techniques to ease her progression through labor. According to the Gate-Control theory, which stimuli could be used to block transmission of the painful stimuli during a contraction?
    1. Focusing on a focal point.
    2. Listening to relaxation music.
    3. Using effleurage.
    4. Engaging in hypnosis.

62. Correct answer - 3. Effleurage is rhythmic circles over the abdomen during contractions. This lets cutaneous stimulation block impulses of painful contraction impulses. Option 1: A focal point would be a visual stimulation. Option 2: Listening to music is an auditory stimulation. Option 4: Hypnosis is an auditory stimulation.
CN: Physiological integrity

63. A primigravida client is having a prolonged second stage of labor. Her health care provider asks for the vacuum extractor to shorten the second stage. What is the most common potential complication for the newborn in this type of delivery?
    1. Caput succedaneum
    2. Prolapsed cord
    3. Asphyxia
    4. Fractured clavicle

64. A 10-week pregnant client comes to the clinic with persistent vomiting, poor skin turgor, and increased pulse rate. She is admitted with a diagnosis of hyperemesis gravidarum. What are the *best initial* diet orders for her?
    1. Six small dry feedings daily
    2. 1 ounce of water offered hourly
    3. Low-fat soft diet as tolerated
    4. NPO

65. A primigravida who is 10 weeks pregnant calls the nurse at the clinic to report that she is experiencing slight vaginal bleeding and pelvic cramps. Which of these instructions by the nurse is *most* appropriate at this time?
    1. "Save any perineal pads, clots, or tissue and come to the clinic right away."
    2. "Lie down on your left side and call again if the flow increases."
    3. "Avoid exercise and sexual intercourse for the next 2 weeks."
    4. "A slight discharge is normal at the time of the month that you would have normally menstruated."

63. Correct answer - 1. Because of the negative pressure from a vacuum extraction, a newborn will be born with a caput and sometimes also a cephalhematoma. Option 2: Vacuum extraction is done when the head has fully engaged and there is no cord prolapse. Option 3: Vacuum extraction is done to prevent asphyxia caused by prolonged second stage. Option 4: There may be a rare instance that an infant would have a caput and fractured clavicle, but this is because of shoulder dystocia.
CN: Physiological integrity

64. Correct answer - 4. For at least the first 24 hours, the client should be NPO with 3,000 ml of I.V. fluids infused. Option 1: This will be later in her dietary regimen. Option 2: The client needs to be NPO for 24 hours first. Option 3: This is the diet the client will be taught to follow when discharged.
CN: Safe, effective care environment

65. Correct answer - 1. Bleeding is a danger sign in pregnancy and may indicate a threatened abortion, especially with cramping. The client should be examined promptly to determine the cause of bleeding. Option 2: The client need not lie on the left side. Option 3: After examination, and with slight bleeding, the client may be prescribed bed rest, abstinence from coitus, and perhaps sedation. If bleeding stops, she may undertake limited activities. Option 4: Once it is determined that a client is pregnant, it is not normal to have bleeding at any time.
CN: Health promotion and maintenance

66. The nurse assesses the fundus of a woman who is 1 day postpartum and finds the following:
    Uterus firm, deviated to the right, and located one finger-breadth below the umbilicus
    Lochia rubra, moderate
    Based on these findings, which action should the nurse take?
    1. Check the woman's pulse and blood pressure.
    2. Encourage the woman to void.
    3. Massage the woman's fundus.
    4. Notify the nurse in charge.

66. Correct answer - 2. When a woman's uterus is deviated to right, it is frequently because of a full bladder. Therefore, option 2 is correct. There is no need to take the actions suggested by options 1, 3, and 4.
    CN: Health promotion and maintenance

67. A client is being discharged from the hospital following evacuation of a hydatidiform mole. The *most* important teaching for this client is to
    1. not get pregnant for 1 year.
    2. seek genetic counseling for future pregnancies.
    3. not get pregnant again.
    4. get RhoGAM immediately, with her next pregnancy.

67. Correct answer - 1. This client must not get pregnant for 1 year after a hydatiform mole because of the high risk of choriocarcinoma development. Option 2: Genetic counseling is not necessary post hydatiform mole. Option 3: This client can become pregnant again, but should wait a minimum of 1 year. Option 4: This is not a problem due to RhoGAM.
    CN: Health promotion and maintenance

68. A woman who is a primigravida is in the 22nd week of her pregnancy. The nurse should expect the fundus of the woman's uterus to be located
    1. at the level of the symphysis pubis.
    2. three finger-breadths above the umbilicus.
    3. one finger-breadth below the xiphoid.
    4. at the level of the umbilicus.

68. Correct answer - 4. At 20 to 24 weeks, the fundus is located at the umbilus. Option 1: At 12 weeks, the fundus is located at the symphysis pubis. Option 2: At 28 weeks, the fundus is three finger-breadths above the umbilicus. Option 3: The fundus moves upward until the 36th week, when it is at the level of the xiphoid.
    CN: Health promotion and maintenance

69. A multigravida in her 30th week of pregnancy is admitted to the hospital with a diagnosis of severe pregnancy-induced hypertension (PIH). The woman is started on magnesium sulfate therapy. While she is on the medication, the nurse should check her
    1. deep tendon reflexes.
    2. blood glucose levels.
    3. urine for acetone.
    4. for bronchospasms.

69. Correct answer - 1. Magnesium sulfate is a central nervous system depressant that is used to prevent seizures. Early indications of magnesium toxicity include depressed deep tendon reflexes. Options 2 and 3: Although it is necessary to check for adequate urinary output, there is no need to check for acetone in the urine or changes in blood glucose levels. Option 4: Since magnesium toxicity may lead to respiratory depression or paralysis, checking the rate of respirations is important but not for the presence of bronchospasms.
CN: Safe, effective care environment

70. A multipara is 1 day postpartum after delivering a 10-pound (4,536-gm) baby. Since the baby was large for gestational age, this woman should be observed for
    1. a urinary tract infection.
    2. signs of hypertension.
    3. decreased lochial flow.
    4. uterine atony.

70. Correct answer - 4. When a woman has had many children or large babies, her uterus may have difficulty contracting. If there is uterine atony, hemorrhage and subsequent hypotension may occur. Therefore, options 2 and 3 are incorrect. Option 1 is incorrect.
CN: Health promotion and maintenance

HOW TO SCORE AND USE THE DIAGNOSTIC PROFILE

In the top "QUESTION NUMBER" row of boxes, mark each question number you answered wrong. Under each question number, check the box in the "TEST TAKING SKILLS" section that is the most appropriate reason you answered the question incorrectly. Do the same for the "CLIENT NEED CATEGORIES" section. The client need category code follows the rationale. Total the number of check marks, by line, in the "Totals" column. This provides you with a profile of your weak areas that should be improve upon prior to taking the NCLEX-RN.

PERSONAL DIAGNOSTIC PROFILE

QUESTION NUMBER																				Totals
TEST-TAKING SKILLS																				
Misread the question																				
Missed important point																				
Forgot fact or concept																				
Applied wrong fact or concept																				
Drew wrong conclusion																				
Incorrectly evaluated distractors																				
Mistakenly selected answer choice																				
Read into question																				
Made a wrong guess																				
Misunderstood question																				
CLIENT NEED CATEGORIES																				
Safe, effective care environment																				
Physiological integrity																				
Psychosocial integrity																				
Health promotion and maintenance																				

CALCULATION OF SUBSCORES

After you score your test, determine your subscores in these client need categories by filling in the following grid.

CLIENT NEED

	Safe, effective care environment	Physiological integrity	Psychosocial integrity	Health promotion & maintenance
Number of questions	10	30	0	30
Number incorrect				
Number correct				
Percent correct*				

*To determine the percent correct in each category, divide the number of items answered correctly by the total number of items and multiply the result by 100.

Note: This is a short test with a limited sample of items in each category. Therefore, if a score in any category is less than 75% correct, further study is strongly advised.

CHAPTER 7

Post-test

Purpose
The Post-test is designed to evaluate your ability to apply nursing principles to a variety of clients. These principles are likely to be tested on NCLEX-RN.

Instructions
This Post-test consists of 90 individual questions. Each question is followed by four possible answers. Read each question and all possible answers carefully, then select the *one* best answer. Remember, each question has only *one* correct answer.

Circle the option you select.

After you've completed the test, check your responses against the correct answers. The correct answers, as well as rationale for correct and incorrect options, are provided immediately following this test. The major purpose of comparing your answers to the test questions with the answer key is to provide further guidance for studying before NCLEX-RN. Each question in the Post-test is coded with the client need category (CN) and the clinical area (CA). The codes follow the rationale.

For the items that you answered correctly, review the rationale to make sure you got the right answer for the right *reason*. For items that you answered incorrectly, read the rationale and determine the reason why you choose an incorrect option. Was it because you didn't know the content or was it because you marked an answer incorrectly by mistake?

After you have looked at each of the rationales, complete the Personal Diagnostic Profile at the end of the answers and calculate the subscrores. Evaluate your overall performance on the test. If you got scores below 75% in a category, review content related to that category.

1. Until the patency of an infant's esophagus can be determined, the nurse should withhold the first feeding of an infant who is born with a maternal history of which of these conditions?
   1. Polyhydramnios
   2. Hyperemesis gravidarum
   3. Pregnancy-induced hypertension
   4. Gestational carbohydrate intolerance

2. A client hospitalized under a voluntary admission has a diagnosis of paranoid schizophrenia. He tells the nurse that he wants to make a telephone call to his lawyer concerning a lawsuit that he initiated against his former health care provider. The nurse should take which of these actions?
   1. Ask the client what the lawsuit is about.
   2. Call the lawyer to explain that the client is hospitalized.
   3. Let the client make the call without seeking further information.
   4. Tell the client that he must discuss the matter with his psychiatrist before making a call.

3. A 28-year-old female client from the West Indies wears numerous silver bracelets or "bangles" on both wrists. When asked to remove them, she refuses. The nurse should recognize that the client's refusal may be related to the cultural belief that the bangles
   1. assure the wearer's fertility.
   2. demonstrate the wearer's/family's wealth or success.
   3. protect the wearer from evil forces or spirits.
   4. enhance the wearer's feminine beauty.

4. A client is admitted to the hospital because of a suspected myocardial infarction (MI). An elevation in which of these blood tests would help to confirm the diagnosis?
   1. Lactic acid
   2. Cholinesterase
   3. Triglycerides
   4. Creatine phosphokinase

5. Which of these measures should be included in the care of a client who is getting oxygen therapy by nasal cannula?
   1. Lubricate the client's nares with petroleum jelly every shift.
   2. Keep the cannula tubing taped to the client's cheeks.
   3. Check that the client's oxygen is being humidified.
   4. Remove the oxygen when the client is eating.

6. The nurse has instructed a client about the use of a diaphragm for contraception. Learning will have occurred if the client plans to leave the device in place for how many hours following coitus?
   1. 2 to 4
   2. 6 to 8
   3. 10 to 12
   4. 14 to 16

7. A 3-month-old infant who has had diarrhea has reddened and excoriated areas on his buttocks. In addition to keeping the areas clean and dry, which of these measures should be included in his care?
   1. Apply a bland lotion to the involved area.
   2. Expose the involved area to light and air.
   3. Use cloth diapers only.
   4. Use sterile disposable diapers only.

8. A newborn infant is suspected of having an esophageal atresia with a tracheoesophageal fistula. He should be assessed for the presence of
   1. difficulty swallowing.
   2. excessive drooling.
   3. projectile vomiting.
   4. sternal retraction.

9. A client in preterm labor at 32-weeks gestation is getting ritodrine hydrochloride (Yutopar) by I.V. infusion. She should be observed for adverse effects, which include
   1. tinnitus
   2. hypoglycemia
   3. tachycardia
   4. hyperkalemia

Page 150

10. A 3-month-old infant has a plaster of Paris hip-spica cast applied for the treatment of a developmental hip dysplasia. While the cast is drying, the nursing diagnosis that should be given the *highest* priority is risk for
    1. pain related to musculoskeletal injury.
    2. sensorimotor activity deficit related to limited physical activity.
    3. impaired skin integrity related to irritation from cast.
    4. altered peripheral tissue perfusion related to cast constriction.

11. An 84-year-old resident in a long-term care facility is terminally ill with metastatic cancer. He has signed a living will, and his family has agreed that no extraordinary means will be used to prolong his life. The resident is unconscious and death is imminent. Several family members arrive at the facility. The nurse informs them about the resident's condition. Which of these interventions with the family would be *most* appropriate?
    1. Ask the family if they would like to go to the resident's bedside for a last visit.
    2. Escort the family to a private conference room where they can wait until the resident's death is pronounced.
    3. Inform the family that the resident is not aware of what is going on around him.
    4. Tell the family to go home as there is nothing more that they can do for him.

12. A paraplegic client has been in the hospital for a month for treatment of a spinal fracture at the second thoracic vertebra. He suddenly complains of a severe pounding headache and nasal congestion. He is sweating profusely and has bradycardia. His blood pressure has risen suddenly. Given these data, the nurse should get the answer to which of these questions?
    1. What is the stimulus that has triggered this episode in the client?
    2. Has the client developed essential hypertension?
    3. When was the last time that the client ate?
    4. Does the client need to drink a sweetened beverage right away?

13. A client who has type 1 (insulin dependent) diabetes is scheduled for major surgery at 10 a.m. The client has been receiving isophane (NPH) insulin and Regular insulin at 7 a.m. The health care provider is not available. Which of these actions would be appropriate?
    1. Give half the prescribed dose of each insulin.
    2. Give prescribed dose of NPH insulin.
    3. Give prescribed dose of regular Insulin.
    4. Withhold the insulins from the client.

14. When a nurse makes an error in documentation on a client's chart, which of these actions should she take?
    1. Draw a single line through the error, mark "error," and initial.
    2. Cover the error with white-out erasure fluid, mark "error," and initial.
    3. Black out the error with a pen, mark "written in error," and initial.
    4. Place brackets around the error, mark "written in error," and initial.

15. A client is admitted to the hospital in Addisonian crisis. An *immediate* goal is to
    1. improve electrolyte balance.
    2. reduce the volume of circulating fluids.
    3. stimulate activity of the adrenal medulla.
    4. depress secretion of corticosteroids.

16. The nurse learns that a prenatal client has a digestive intolerance to lactose. The client's plan of care should be modified to ensure an adequate intake of which of these nutrients?
    1. Folic acid
    2. Thiamine
    3. Iron
    4. Calcium

17. A client is admitted to hospital because of a cerebrovascular accident. She is unconscious. Her care plan includes all of the following nursing diagnoses. Which one should get *priority* in her care?
    1. Sensory/perceptual alteration related to unconsciousness
    2. Impaired physical mobility related to unconsciousness
    3. Altered nutrition: less than body requirements related to unconsciousness
    4. Ineffective airway clearance related to unconsciousness

18. A client who has severe diarrhea should be assessed for the development of
    1. metabolic acidosis.
    2. respiratory acidosis.
    3. metabolic alkalosis.
    4. respiratory alkalosis.

19. A 3-year-old boy, who is to get prednisone (Deltasone) orally, weighs 33 pounds. The order for his Deltasone is 2mg/kg of body weight, to be given in evenly divided doses daily. The boy should get how many mg of Deltasone in a 24-hour period?
    1. 15
    2. 30
    3. 45
    4. 60

20. Which statement by a client who is on long-term therapy with chlorpromazine hydrochloride (Thorazine) indicates a need for *further* instruction about the drug's effects?
    1. "I will take a cold medicine if I get any signs of a cold."
    2. "I shouldn't stay out in the sun for long."
    3. "I will make sure there is plenty of roughage in my diet."
    4. "I shouldn't sit for a long time in a hot bath."

21. A1-month-old infant is being treated for developmental hip dysplasia with a Pavlik harness. The infant's mother should be given which of these instructions about the infant's care during this treatment?
    1. "Keep him in the supine position when in bed."
    2. "Measure the girth of his thighs each morning."
    3. "Remove the device every 4 hours for 1 hour and exercise his legs."
    4. "Check his skin under the device for irritation every day."

22. A 2-year-old child with a diagnosis of Hirschsprung's disease has a rectal biopsy. The mother asks the nurse, "What is the purpose of the biopsy?" The nurse should respond that the purpose of the biopsy is to determine if
    1. excessive proliferation of normal cells is present.
    2. atrophic changes are occurring in the cells.
    3. autonomic parasympathetic ganglion cells are absent.
    4. genetic engineering is a feasible solution.

23. A nurse instructor is helping a student nurse prepare to give an adult client 3 ml of an ordered drug intramuscularly. Prior to administering the drug, the nurse asks the student nurse to describe the steps in the procedure. The student nurse's description includes all of the following statements. For which one should the nurse get additional information because it is *incorrect*?
    1. "I'll use a 21 gauge, 1½-inch needle for the injection."
    2. "I'm going to use the deltoid muscle for the injection site."
    3. "I'll put some ice on the injection site before injecting the medication."
    4. "I'm going to inject the needle at a 90-degree angle into the skin."

24. A client who is hospitalized for pulmonary emphysema is having difficulty raising thick respiratory secretions. To help the client, which of these instructions would be *best?*
    1. "Try to drink nine or ten glasses of fluid a day."
    2. "When you're in bed, make sure you turn from side to side every hour."
    3. "Breathe through pursed lips four or five times every hour."
    4. "Take several deep breaths before you cough."

25. A client is admitted to the coronary care unit with the diagnosis of MI. The client tells the nurse, "My health care provider says that I had a heart attack, but I think it was just indigestion from the pizza I ate yesterday." The nurse should recognize that the client is using which of these defense mechanisms?
    1. Rationalization
    2. Regression
    3. Displacement
    4. Denial

26. A client who has Parkinson's disease is likely to have which of these symptoms?
    1. Dry, translucent skin
    2. Masklike facial expression
    3. Excessive tearing of the eyes
    4. Flaccid upper extremities at rest

27. On the second postoperative day, a client who has had a craniotomy begins to secrete clear drainage from the nose. The client has been receiving dexamethasone (Decadron). Based on these findings, it would be *most* important for the nurse to get the answer to which of these questions?
    1. When was the last time the client blew his nose?
    2. Has the client experienced an adverse effect of Decadron?
    3. Does the client's drainage contain glucose?
    4. Is the client developing a cold?

28. A nurse is conducting a chart audit of a 2-year-old boy who has nephrotic syndrome. Because he has massive generalized edema, the nurse should expect that which of these measures is being included in his care?
    1. Maintaining him in a side-lying position.
    2. Massaging his skin with an astringent.
    3. Applying elastic bandages to his legs.
    4. Supporting his scrotum on a soft pad.

29. A nurse is speaking to parents about tuberculosis (TB) at the local school district meeting. Which of these facts should the nurse give to the parents about TB?
    1. It is important that a natural resistance to TB be maintained by proper nutrition and rest.
    2. It is essential that all school-aged children be tested for TB twice a year.
    3. It has been proven that children under age 4 have a natural immunity to TB.
    4. It is scientifically documented that pyridoxine hydrochloride supplements act as a barrier to the TB bacteria.

30. A client is brought to the emergency department with a tentative diagnosis of acute pulmonary edema. Which action should be taken *first?*
    1. Elevate the client's lower extremities.
    2. Attach the client to a cardiac monitor.
    3. Check that the client is in high-Fowler's position.
    4. Start an I.V. infusion on the client.

31. A client who is being treated for myxedema is given instructions about her care. Which of these comments indicates that she has understood the instructions?
    1. "My disease makes me more sensitive to heat."
    2. "I will have to have an operation to remove my thyroid gland."
    3. "I will have to take medicine for the rest of my life."
    4. "At least I'll never have to worry about gaining weight."

32. A client is being observed for symptoms of chronic open-angle glaucoma, which include
    1. gradual loss of color perception.
    2. gradual decrease in visual acuity.
    3. seeing moving spots or floaters.
    4. seeing halos around bright lights.

33. A nurse on a mental health unit has been interacting daily with a client with a goal of establishing a therapeutic relationship. Which of these behaviors, if exhibited by the client, would indicate that the relationship had entered the working phase?
    1. Asking the nurse what to expect from the relationship.
    2. Addressing the nurse using the nurse's first name.
    3. Expressing sadness that the relationship will end.
    4. Initiating contact with the nurse to discuss an issue.

34. A client had a modified radical mastectomy 3 days ago. Her dressing has just been changed and her drainage tubes removed. She states to the nurse, "Did you see my huge, red incision and the holes left from the drains? It looks horrible!"
    Which of these responses by the nurse would be appropriate?
    1. "Your incision is inflamed now, but in several weeks the redness and swelling will decrease and the skin will look much better."
    2. "Although it's difficult, you must be strong and learn to accept and cope with the changed appearance of your body."
    3. "Your incision actually looks very good, considering the extensive surgery that was performed."
    4. "You must be concerned about how other people will react to the change in your appearance."

35. A staff member who is apparently intoxicated reports for duty on the pediatric unit. Which of these actions would be appropriate for the nurse to take *initially?*
    1. Send the staff member home.
    2. Advise the staff member to seek help from Alcoholic Anonymous.
    3. Assign the staff member to non-client care tasks.
    4. Discuss the staff member's condition with a supervisor.

36. A 15-month-old girl with iron-deficiency anemia is to get supplements in the form of liquid ferrous sulfate (Feosol). The charge nurse can determine that the mother is using the correct procedure to administer the Feosol if the mother is giving it to her from a
    1. medicine dropper, placed well back on her tongue.
    2. small cup, pouring a small amount of the medication at a time in back of her lower teeth.
    3. syringe, squirting the medication into one side of her mouth.
    4. plastic spoon, put between her lips.

37. An infant born with a cleft palate is to be sent home to await corrective surgery when he is 8 months old. The nurse can determine that the infant's parents understood the discharge teaching correctly if they make which comment?
    1. "We will delay our baby's immunizations until after the operation."
    2. "We will keep our baby from lying on his stomach."
    3. "We will use a variety of methods to feed our baby."
    4. "We'll call our health care provider if our baby gets a cold."

38. The nurse is assessing a client for symptoms of a spastic bladder, which include
    1. urgency.
    2. nocturia.
    3. reflexive emptying of the bladder.
    4. increased contractions of the bladder muscle.

39. A nurse has given a client instructions in preparation for a myelogram. The client will get an oil-based contrast medium for the test. The client has understood the instructions if he makes which of these comments?
    1. "My groin will be shaved before the test."
    2. "The x-ray table will be tilted in various positions during the test."
    3. "I will have to hold my breath periodically during the test."
    4. "I will have to sit upright in bed for several hours after the test."

40. A 4-year-old girl with acute lymphocytic leukemia (ALL) has a platelet count of 30,000/mm^3. Because of this information, the nursing care plan at this time should include which of these notations?
    1. "Avoid forceful nose blowing."
    2. "Provide a diet high in vitamin C."
    3. "Test urine for pH q.i.d."
    4. "Discontinue live vaccine immunizations."

41. The nurse is to give digoxin (Lanoxin) to a 3-year-old girl with a congenital heart defect. The girl's apical pulse rate is 90 bpm. Which of these actions should the nurse take next?
    1. Give the Lanoxin to the girl as ordered.
    2. Give one-half the ordered dose of Lanoxin to the girl.
    3. Wait 1 hour and retake the apical pulse before giving the Lanoxin to the girl.
    4. Notify the girl's health care provider and discuss the Lanoxin order.

42. A client who is 28 weeks pregnant tells the nurse, "I had to have my rings cut off because my hands were so puffy." Based on this data, the nurse should seek additional information concerning the
    1. height of the fundus.
    2. fetal heart rate.
    3. presence of protein in the urine.
    4. presence of human placental lactogen in the blood.

43. After a kidney transplant 3 days earlier, a client has oliguria, a temperature of 102.2° F (39° C) and tenderness over the graft site. Based on these findings, the nurse should, *initially,* suspect that the client has which of these conditions?
    1. Acute kidney failure
    2. Cystitis
    3. Graft rejection
    4. Urinary tract obstruction

44. A client who has just been diagnosed as having pulmonary TB is started on anti-tuberculosis drugs in the outpatient clinic. Before the client goes home, which of these instructions should he be given?
    1. "You won't be able to return to your job as a manager until the course of drug therapy is completed."
    2. "You will need to take your drugs until five successive sputum specimens are negative."
    3. "Use disposable eating utensils and paper plates when eating with your family."
    4. "Cover your mouth and nose with double-ply tissue when you cough or sneeze."

45. A client is 20 weeks pregnant. At this stage of pregnancy, the nurse should expect the uterine fundus to be palpable at the level of which of these anatomical landmarks?
    1. Symphysis pubis
    2. Umbilicus
    3. Costal margins
    4. Xiphoid process

46. A newborn infant of a mother with type 1(insulin-dependent) diabetes is admitted to the nursery. Because the infant's mother has diabetes, his care plan should include monitoring for which of these potential problems?
    1. Anemia
    2. Hypoglycemia
    3. Hypercalcemia
    4. Hyperphosphatemia

47. A 17-year-old boy is lighting the grill at a family picnic when the sleeve of his shirt goes up in flames. His sister, who is a nurse, puts out the flames. Which of these actions would be appropriate for her to take *next?*
    1. Remove her brother's shirt from the burned areas.
    2. Place a blanket over her brother.
    3. Put cold water over her brother's burned areas.
    4. Have her brother assume a supine position.

48. A client on an inpatient psychiatric unit claims that she gets divine revelations through a special microchip God placed in her brain. On the unit, she walks around, mumbling to herself, stopping occasionally to "bestow God's blessing" on clients and staff members. Which of these approaches should be included in the client's plan of care?
    1. Encourage the client to verbalize the content of the divine revelations.
    2. Assign the client homework of selected Bible readings and their interpretations.
    3. Explain to the client that her beliefs could not possibly be true.
    4. Maintain the client's focus on one reality-based activity at a time.

49. A depressed female client on an inpatient psychiatric unit refuses to get out of bed to bathe and dress. The window shades are drawn and her room is completely dark. She states, "What's the use? I'm no good to anyone. Don't bother with me." Which of these actions by the nurse is *best?*
    1. Tell her the nurse cares and thinks she is worthwhile.
    2. Let her stay in bed and try to get her up later.
    3. Kindly but firmly help her bathe and dress.
    4. Silently remain with the client in the darkened room.

50. A client has been treated for Addison's disease. She is admitted to the hospital in Addisonian crisis. Which of these comments, if made by the client, would *most* clearly identify the possible precipitating cause for the crisis?
    1. "I've had the flu for a couple of days."
    2. "I've been adding extra salt to my food because it's been so hot and humid."
    3. "I took an extra prednisone tablet this morning."
    4. "I'm expecting my menstrual period today."

51. A client is scheduled for surgery. The evening before the scheduled surgery, the nurse observes that the results of the client's blood tests include all of the following values. Which one should be reported to the health care provider *immediately* because it may cause the surgery to be cancelled?
    1. Hemoglobin, 13 g/dl
    2. Hematocrit, 46%
    3. Total protein, 6 g/dl
    4. Blood urea nitrogen, 42 g/dl

52. When admitting a 16-year-old boy who has cystic fibrosis (CF) to the hospital for treatment of bacterial pneumonia, the nurse should *definitely* get the answer to which of these questions?
    1. Has he cut his wisdom teeth yet?
    2. Does he limit his sugar intake?
    3. Can he or another responsible person in his household administer I.V. antibiotics?
    4. How often does he do prophylactic chest physical therapy?

53. Following a lobectomy, the nurse should passively exercise the client's arm on the operative side to prevent
    1. osteoarthritis.
    2. synovitis.
    3. frozen shoulder.
    4. elbow tendonitis.

54. Which of these nursing diagnoses should be given priority in the care of a client who has acute pulmonary edema and is on bed rest?
    1. Risk for impaired skin integrity related to edema and bed rest.
    2. Altered tissue perfusion related to decreased blood flow to tissues and edema.
    3. Activity intolerance related to imbalance between oxygen supply and demand.
    4. Risk for knowledge deficit related to self-care activities.

55. A postpartum client is planning to breast-feed. To keep the nipples in good condition for breast-feeding and to prevent infection, which of these measures should the nurse include in the client's care plan?
    1. Washing the nipples with soap and water before each feeding.
    2. Exposing the nipples to air and sunlight for short periods of time.
    3. Using a plastic bra liner to handle leakage.
    4. Cleansing the nipples with a mild antiseptic solution.

56. A newborn is admitted to the high-risk nursery after a precipitate birth in the car on the way to the hospital. The infant was exposed to very cold weather and is placed in a radiant warmer. Given these data, the nurse should seek additional information by asking which of these questions?
    1. Is the infant shivering?
    2. Are the infant's hands and feet cyanotic?
    3. Are the infant's fontanels soft?
    4. Is the infant experiencing apnea?

57. A nurse working in a prenatal clinic learns that some of the clients practice pica. Clients who practice pica during pregnancy should be assessed for which of these conditions?
    1. Anemia
    2. Hydramnios
    3. Diabetes mellitus
    4. Multiple pregnancy

58. Recently, in one nurse's community, there have been several suicide attempts by high school students. Which of these behaviors should she recognize as a danger signal for suicide among adolescents?
    1. Inability to communicate with parents.
    2. Preoccupation with personal appearance.
    3. Spending long periods with close friends.
    4. Intense involvement in school activities outside the classroom.

59. The nurse is performing a mental status examination on a physically stable, 72-year-old client who recently moved to a life-care community. Which of these questions should the nurse ask to evaluate the client's judgment?
    1. "How many pennies are in two dollars?"
    2. "How are a bird and a butterfly alike?"
    3. "What is the meaning of, 'A rolling stone gathers no moss'?"
    4. "What would you do if you entered your apartment and smelled gas?"

60. A 2-year-old is admitted to the hospital with acute laryngotracheobronchitis. All of the following goals are developed for the baby. The *priority* goal, during the acute phase, should be to
    1. provide optimum nutrition.
    2. conserve energy.
    3. maintain skin integrity.
    4. provide sensory stimulation.

61. A client with pulmonary TB is given a prescription for isoniazid (INH) and rifampin (Rifadin). The client says to the nurse, "Why do I need to take two medications? Can't one cure my TB?" Which of these responses by the nurse is accurate?
    1. "Rifadin increases the potency of INH."
    2. "INH stimulates Rifadin to penetrate the cytoplasm of the tubercle bacilli."
    3. "Both drugs are given together in case the tubercle bacilli become resistant to one."
    4. "Both drugs counteract each other's adverse effects."

62. A common adverse effect of diphtheria, tetanus, and pertussis (DPT) vaccine given to an infant would *most* likely be manifested by which of these symptoms?
    1. Vomiting
    2. Hematuria
    3. Sudden elevated temperature
    4. Swelling at the injection site

63. A homeless man with a dual diagnosis of schizophrenia and substance abuse is admitted to the inpatient unit after making obscene remarks and threatening gestures to people on the street. He tells the nurse that "voices" have been telling him to protect himself from "enemies" who want to kill him. On the unit, the client is tense and pacing. All of the following nursing diagnoses have been made for the client. Which one should have *priority?*
    1. Social isolation related to inability to trust.
    2. Sensory-perceptual alteration related to stress.
    3. Risk for violence related to auditory hallucinations.
    4. Ineffective individual coping related to an inadequate support system.

64. An 84-year-old man was recently admitted to a life-care facility. He tells the nurse that he is having difficulty sleeping at night. To promote sleep, which of these actions should the nurse take?
    1. Request a sedative to be administered to the client nightly.
    2. Encourage the client to take a daily afternoon nap.
    3. Help the client establish a bedtime routine.
    4. Limit the client's activity during the day.

65. An infant is being observed for symptoms of pyloric stenosis, which include
    1. foul smelling, fatty stools.
    2. excessive salivation.
    3. poor sucking response.
    4. projectile vomiting.

66. The health care provider orders neomycin sulfate (Mycifradin) orally for a client with severe cirrhosis of the liver. The therapeutic effect of the drug for this client would be achieved if he had a *decrease* in which of these blood levels?
    1. Creatinine
    2. Acid phosphatase
    3. Ammonia
    4. Haptoglobin

67. A client undergoing detoxification from alcohol should be observed for withdrawal symptoms, which include
    1. hyperglycemia.
    2. hypertension.
    3. hypouricemia.
    4. hypothermia.

68. A client who has chronic renal failure is getting hemodialysis treatments. Her orders also include aluminum hydroxide (Amphojel) on a daily basis. A student nurse asks a staff nurse if the Amphojel should be discontinued because the client denies that she has gastric distress. The staff nurse's response should include that the purpose of the Amphojel for the client is to
    1. promote the excretion of potassium.
    2. reduce serum phosphate levels.
    3. minimize the transport of sodium across the sodium pump.
    4. enhance the absorption of magnesium.

69. A client who has a cerebrovascular accident is being treated with I.V. heparin sodium (Liquaemin sodium). The medication has achieved its intended effect if the results of her blood tests indicate that her
    1. prothrombin time is between 1½ and 2½ times the normal control level.
    2. prothrombin time is between 3 and 4 times the normal control level.
    3. partial thromboplastin time is between 1½ and 2½ times the normal control level.
    4. partial thromboplastin time is between 3 and 4 times the normal control level.

70. Following a bronchoscopy, a female client has all of the following symptoms. The nurse should *definitely* collect additional data about which one because it may indicate that the client is developing a complication of the test?
    1. She has a headache.
    2. She has slightly blood-tinged sputum.
    3. She is dyspneic.
    4. She is belching.

71. A 3-month-old-male infant who had developmental dysplasia of his right hip has had a corrective procedure. Which of these findings would indicate that the procedure has corrected the infant's defect?
    1. The infant is able to fully abduct his affected extremity.
    2. The circumference of the infant's thighs are equal in size.
    3. The infant is able to turn more easily from side to side.
    4. The femoral pulse is palpable on the infant's affected side.

72. Because of an adverse effect of furosemide (Lasix), a client who is getting high doses of the medication should be instructed to
    1. rise slowly from a lying or sitting position.
    2. eliminate tyramine-containing foods from his diet.
    3. limit the intake of oral fluids to 1,000 ml daily.
    4. check the apical pulse before administration.

73. After having a suprapubic prostatectomy a client is being prepared for discharge. Which of these statements by the client indicates that he has understood the instructions?
    1. "I can engage in sexual intercourse in about 3 weeks."
    2. "I may dribble urine for several months."
    3. "I'll be able to start my cross-country motor trip in three weeks as planned."
    4. "I should wait until my bladder is really full before voiding for the next month."

74. A client who is being treated for chronic open-angle glaucoma is scheduled for an abdominal hysterectomy. Her preoperative preparation includes all of the following orders. Which one should the nurse *definitely* question?
    1. Standard abdominal preparation and shave on the evening before surgery.
    2. Vaginal douche with tap water on the evening before surgery.
    3. Meperidine (Demerol) hydrochloride 75 mg I.M. on call to the operating room.
    4. Atropine sulfate 0.4 mg I.M. on call to the operating room.

75. A nursing instructor has reviewed the procedure for inserting a nasogastric tube with a student nurse. Which of these statements by the student indicates that *further* instruction is needed?
    1. "The tube should be lubricated with a water-soluble jelly before insertion."
    2. "The client should tilt his head back before the tube is inserted."
    3. "The client should breathe through his mouth as the tube is being inserted."
    4. "The client should cough as the tube is being inserted."

76. A client who has type 1 (insulin-dependent) diabetes mellitus is brought to the emergency department by his family. He is confused and has Kussmaul respirations. He also has a fruity odor to his breath and his blood pressure is 80/50 mm Hg. After examining the client, the health care provider writes all of the following orders. Which one should the nurse *question?*
    1. I.V. #1--1,000 ml 0.9% normal saline to run in over 3 hours.
    2. Add 40 meq potassium chloride to I.V. #1.
    3. I.V. #2--100 units Regular insulin in 1,000 ml 0.9% normal saline to run at 25 ml/hour.
    4. 50 ml of 50% dextrose in water by I.V. push.

77. A depressed client with suicidal ideation is admitted to the psychiatric unit. A tricyclic antidepressant is prescribed. Which of these precautions should be emphasized in the client's care plan?
    1. Check that the client has not ingested food immediately prior to taking the medication.
    2. Limit the client's physical activity until the medication takes effect.
    3. Monitor the client for excessive weight gain.
    4. Be sure that the client swallows the medication.

78. The nurse teaches a client, who is 38 weeks pregnant, how to determine the duration of her contractions when she goes into labor. The instructions have been understood if the client states that she will time from the
    1. beginning of one contraction to the beginning of the next contraction.
    2. beginning of the contraction to the acme of that contraction.
    3. beginning of the contraction to the end of that contraction.
    4. end of one contraction to the beginning of the next contraction.

79. A client has been treated for herion addiction and is entering a methadone maintenance program. In preparing him for methadone maintenance, the teaching plan should include which of the following information?
    1. "Methadone is a non-addictive substitute for heroin."
    2. "Methadone can be administered only by the oral route."
    3. "Withdrawal from methadone is accompanied by few physical symptoms of short duration."
    4. "Methadone does not produce the high that is associated with heroin."

80. A client had a supratentorial craniotomy 3 days ago. On morning rounds, a nurse makes all of the following observations of the client. Which one requires *immediate* correction?
    1. The side rails of the bed are padded.
    2. The head of the bed is flat.
    3. The client is getting oxygen at 5 liters a minute.
    4. The client lying on his non-operative side.

81. To determine if a client is at risk for essential hypertension, the nurse should get the answer to which of these questions?
    1. "How much alcohol do you drink?"
    2. "How often do you exercise?"
    3. "Do you eat foods that are high in purines?"
    4. "Do you suffer from migraine headaches?"

82. A nurse is preparing a client for an exercise electrocardiograph (stress test). The nurse should assess if the client knows that the purpose of the test is to evaluate the
    1. cardiovascular response to an increased workload.
    2. exact timing and characteristics of extra heart sounds.
    3. cardiac structure and mobility, especially the valves.
    4. pump effectiveness and tissue perfusion.

83. At a well-baby clinic, the nurse should plan to administer the first dose of vaccine for measles, mumps and rubella (MMR) to a child at which of these ages?
    1. 2 months.
    2. 15 months.
    3. 3 years.
    4. 6 years.

84. A mother asks the nurse what causes the respiratory symptoms in her child who has CF. The nurse should explain that the respiratory symptoms are due to
    1. an allergic hypersensitivity to inhaled substances.
    2. abnormally thick, tenacious mucus in the bronchioles.
    3. an inflammation of the pulmonary parenchyma.
    4. increased oxygen-carbon dioxide exchange at the alveoli.

85. The nurse teaches pregnant clients how to do prenatal exercises. Which of these instructions accurately describes Kegel's exercises?
    1. "Tighten the muscle that you would use to stop the flow of urine. Hold for the count of three, then relax the muscle."
    2. "Stand with your back against a wall. Tighten your abdominal muscles and flatten your lower back against the wall."
    3. "Place your thumbs opposite each other near the edge of the areola. Then press into the breast and stretch outward."
    4. "Sit on the floor in a cross-legged, tailor position. Try to keep your thighs flat on the floor."

86. A client is getting phenytoin (Dilantin). He should be observed for adverse effects, which include
    1. gingival hyperplasia.
    2. metallic taste.
    3. hypoglycemia.
    4. hyperammonia.

87. An 8-year-old girl is being prepared for a lumbar puncture. Which one of these measures should be included in her care?
    1. Placing her on NPO for 4 hours before the test.
    2. Telling her that she will have to stay immobile during the test.
    3. Applying a compression dressing to her puncture site after the test.
    4. Checking the specific gravity of her urine for 24 hours after the test.

88. A client has had a subtotal thyroidectomy. Which of these findings might indicate the development of thyroid storm?
    1. Body temperature of 104° F (40° C).
    2. Heart rate of 92 bpm.
    3. Respiratory rate of 22/minute
    4. Blood pressure of 110/60 mm Hg.

89. A client is to get sucralfate (Carafate). The medication is prescribed for which of these purposes?
    1. To stimulate the secretion of pepsin from the gastric mucosa.
    2. To form a protective paste over the gastric mucosa.
    3. To reduce the emptying time of the stomach.
    4. To neutralize hydrochloric acid in the stomach.

90. A client who had peritonitis had a surgical resection 2 days ago. If he made all of the following comments, which one should be investigated *immediately?*
    1. "My stomach is growling."
    2. "I feel as if something just gave way."
    3. "I have been passing a lot of gas."
    4. "My stomach feels soft."

THE CORRECT ANSWERS AND RATIONALE FOLLOW

1. Correct answer - 1. Polyhydramnios is often seen in the maternal history of infants with esophageal atresia because the fetus with an esophageal atresia cannot swallow amniotic fluid. Options 2, 3, and 4: These maternal conditions are not associated with infant conditions that would necessitate withholding feedings to first ensure the patency of the infant's esophagus.
CN: Physiological integrity
CA: Pediatric nursing

2. Correct answer - 3. A client has the right to manage his personal affairs, which includes making telephone calls, sending letters, etc. Options 1 and 4: Asking about the particulars of the lawsuit and referring the client to the

psychiatrist violate this right. Option 2: The nurse's calling the lawyer is a violation of the client's right to privacy.
CN: Safe, effective care environment
CA: Mental health nursing

3. Correct answer - 3. The silver bracelets are open to "let out evil," yet closed to prevent evil from entering the body. Many people believe they are extremely vulnerable to evil, even to death, when these bracelets are removed. Therefore, when these bracelets are removed, the client experiences much anxiety. Options 1, 2, and 4 do not reflect the major purpose of wearing the bracelets.
CN: Safe, effective care environment
CA: Mental health nursing

4. Correct answer - 4. In addition to lactic hydrogenase (LDH) and glutamic-oxaloacetic acid (SGOT), creatine phosphokinase (CPK) is a cardiac enzyme that is used to help establish the diagnosis of MI. When myocardial cells die, these enzymes are released into the bloodstream. The duration of the CPK's elevation is felt to correlate with the extent and severity of the MI. Serum CPK levels increase early--within 6 hours--in myocardial damage; they peak in about 18 hours and return to normal in 3 or 4 days if no further damage occurs. CPK is also found in skeletal muscle and brain cells. Options 1, 2, and 3: Lactic acid is a metabolic intermediate involved in many biochemical processes; cholinesterase is an enzyme that catalyzes the reaction of acetylcholine; and triglycerides are mixtures of two or three fatty acids.
CN: Physiological integrity
CA: Medical/surgical nursing

5. Correct answer - 3. Humidification is required for most forms of oxygen administration. Options 1, 2, and 4: The client's nares should be protected with a water-soluble jelly; the cannula tubing should not be taped to the client's cheek (the elastic portion of the cannula piece should be adjusted so that it fits the client properly); and, the client should get oxygen even while eating.
CN: Safe, effective care environment
CA: Medical/surgical nursing

6. Correct answer - 2. A diaphragm is used with a spermicide and must be kept in place for 6 or 8 hours following intercourse, since it takes 6 hours for the spermicide to destroy the sperm. Option 1: Removing the diaphragm earlier greatly increases the chance of pregnancy. Options 3 and 4: Removing the diaphragm later increases the risk of infection.
CN: Health promotion and maintenance
CA: Maternity nursing

7. Correct answer - 2 . Exposing the buttocks to air and light will speed drying and healing of the area. Options 1, 3, and 4: Lotions are never used when the diaper area is excoriated; the use of cloth or disposable diapers does not make a difference; and sterile diapers are not necessary.
CN: Physiological integrity
CA: Pediatric nursing

8. Correct answer - 2. The presence of esophageal atresia is suspected in an infant with excessive salivation and in a newborn with drooling that is frequently accompanied by choking, coughing, and cyanosis. Options 1, 3, and 4 are not symptoms of this condition.
CN: Physiological integrity
CA: Pediatric nursing

9. Correct answer - 3. A common adverse effect of ritodrine is tachycardia. Options 2, 3, and 4: Other adverse effects include hyperglycemia, rather than hypoglycemia, and hypokalemia, rather than hyperkalemia. Tinnitus is not an adverse effect of ritodrine.
CN: Physiological integrity
CA: Maternity nursing

10. Correct answer - 4. While the cast is drying (the first 24 to 48 hours in an infant this age), the greatest risk is for circulatory compromise because the cast is too tight and tissue edema. Options 1, 2, and 3: Pain and impaired skin integrity may both be the result of impaired peripheral tissue perfusion and therefore are secondary to it in priority at this time. Although sensorimotor activity is important for infants of this age, the integrity of the circulation to casted parts is more important during the initial casting period.

CN: Safe, effective care environment
CA: Pediatric nursing

11. Correct answer - 1. The nurse should offer the family the opportunity to go to the resident's bedside for a final visit. A final visit assists the family in coming to terms with the grieving process and lets the resident know that he is not alone. Options 2 and 4: Placing the family in a conference room or sending them home would prevent this process from occurring. Option 3: Although the resident is unconscious, he may be able to hear and to experience touch.
CN: Health promotion and maintenance
CA: Mental health nursing

12. Correct answer - 1. All of these symptoms indicate that the client is likely experiencing autonomic dysreflexia or autonomic hyperreflexia, which is an acute emergency that occurs as a result of exaggerated responses to stimuli that are not likely to irritate normal individuals. It occurs among clients with cord lesions above the T6 level and generally after spinal shock has subsided. The nurse should assess what has triggered the response in the client (i.e., distended bladder or bowel, draft of cold air). Options 2, 3, and 4: Given the client's history of spinal cord trauma and the suddenness with which the symptoms (especially hypertension) appeared, essential hypertension does not seem likely. Determining the time when the client last ate and his need for a sweetened beverage is irrelevant.
CN: Physiological integrity
CA: Medical/surgical nursing

13. Correct answer - 4. Prior to surgery and many procedures, the health care provider should be consulted to determine if insulin dose(s) should be adjusted. If he is unavailable, hold the insulin. Insulin and glucose intake are carefully controlled for surgical procedures and typically only Regular insulin would be given, although not necessarily the usual dose. Options 1, 2, and 3: The health care provider should always be consulted before medication dosages are adjusted.
CN: Safe, effective care environment
CA: Medical/surgical nursing

14. Correct answer - 1. If an error in documentation is made, the incorrect section should be crossed through with a single line, marked "error," and initialed. Options 2, 3, and 4: Do not erase, apply correction fluid, or scratch out an error made while documenting. The error should not be obliterated so that what was originally written cannot be read.
CN: Safe, effective care environment
CA: Medical/surgical nursing

15. Correct answer - 1. Addisonian crisis is a life-threatening emergency caused by insufficient adrenocortical hormones or a sudden marked decrease in these hormones. As a result, electrolyte imbalances (e.g., hyponatremia and hyperkalemia) occur. These imbalances must be corrected immediately. Options 2, 3, and 4: Clients in Addisonian crisis have fluid volume deficit, which also needs to be corrected immediately. Pathophysiological changes in Addisonian crisis include hyposecretion of hormones from the adrenal cortex (not the adrenal medulla which secretes epinephrine). These clients also have hyposecretion of cortisol, which requires replacement therapy.
CN: Physiological integrity
CA: Medical/surgical nursing

16. Correct answer - 4. Clients with a lactose (milk sugar) intolerance will have inadequate intake of milk and milk products during pregnancy. Therefore, they will need calcium supplements. Options 1, 2, and 3: Milk is not a major source of folic acid, thiamine, or iron.
CN: Health promotion and maintenance
CA: Maternity nursing

17. Correct answer - 4. Although all of these nursing diagnoses are important, priority should be given to ineffective airway clearance because retained respiratory secretions can prove fatal. Such problems can develop in a very short time. Options 1, 2, and 3: All of these nursing diagnoses are associated with complications. However, none are as lethal as ineffective breathing or require constant intervention.
CN: Physiological integrity
CA: Medical/surgical nursing

18. Correct answer - 1. A deficit in bicarbonate ions or an excess in hydrogen ions causes metabolic acidosis. In addition to diarrhea, other causes include shock, excessive dieting, aspirin overdose, uremia, and ketoacidosis. Options 2, 3, and 4 are therefore incorrect. Examples of some conditions associated with these acid-base imbalances are respiratory acidosis (airway obstruction), metabolic alkalosis (excessive vomiting), and respiratory alkalosis (hyperventilation).
CN: Physiological integrity
CA: Medical/surgical nursing

19. Correct answer - 2. To determine how many milligrams the boy should get daily, the first step is to convert his weight in pounds to kilograms (kg). Remember that 1 kg = 2.2 lbs. So,

$$\frac{2.2 \text{ kg.}}{1} = \frac{33 \text{ lbs.}}{x}$$

$$2.2x = 33$$
$$x = 15 \text{ kg}$$

The boy's weight of 33 lbs equals 15 kg. The medication order is for 2 mg/kg of body weight. So, 2 mg x 15 kg = 30 mg. The boy should get 30 mg of the Deltasone in a 24-hour period.
CN: Physiological integrity
CA: Pediatric nursing

20. Correct answer - 1. Many over-the-counter cold medications contain ingredients that have a sedating effect. Combining these preparations with Thorazine can have a profound sedative effect. Options 2, 3, and 4 are appropriate precautions related to Thorazine's adverse effects of photosensitivity, constipation, and orthostatic hypotension.
CN: Psychosocial integrity
CA: Mental health nursing

21. Correct answer - 4. The Pavlik harness places pressure on the skin and is worn at least 23 if not 24 hours per day. Therefore, the infant is a great risk for skin irritation and breakdown on the areas where the device presses on the skin. These areas must be checked daily for signs of irritation and breakdown. Options 1, 2, and 3: The infant can be placed in a variety of positions (e.g., prone, side-lying and even semi-sitting). There is no need to measure thigh girth. The parents should not remove the device unless specifically ordered, and then it would only be for a short time so that they can bathe the infant.
CN: Safe, effective care environment
CA: Pediatric nursing

22. Correct answer - 3. Hirschsprung's disease or aganglionic megacolon occurs when there is an absence of autonomic parasympathetic ganglion cells. Diagnosing aganglionic megacolon usually involves doing a rectal biopsy to determine whether ganglion cells are present. Absence of these nerve cells helps to establish the diagnosis. Options 1, 2, and 4: Because of number 3, these are incorrect.
CN: Safe, effective care environment
CA: Pediatric nursing

23. Correct answer - 2. No more than 2 ml of solution should be administered in the deltoid muscle because the muscle is not well developed in many adults and most children. For adults, one of the gluteal sites (i.e., ventral gluteal or dorsogluteal) is preferred because they are large enough in most adults to have 3 ml of an injection in one site. The gluteal muscles, however, should not be used in children under 3 years old because their muscles are not well developed. Options 1, 3, and 4: These are acceptable for the administration of an I.M. injection.
CN: Safe, effective care environment
CA: Medical/surgical nursing

24. Correct answer - 1. One of the best ways to liquefy thick sputum is to have client drink as much fluid as possible. Options 2, 3, and 4: None of these will help to liquefy secretions.
CN: Physiological integrity
CA: Medical/surgical nursing

25. Correct answer - 4. The client is using denial, refusing to recognize the reality of his disagreeable situation. Option 1: Rationalization refers to finding excuses for one's behavior and ignoring the real reasons for behavior. Option 2: Regression

refers to retreating to behavior characteristic of an earlier level of development. Option 3: Displacement is the transfer of an emotion from one subject or person to another.
CN: Psychosocial integrity
CA: Mental health nursing

26. Correct answer - 2. One of the classic signs of Parkinson's disease is a tremor of the hand, which occurs at rest and may look like a pill-rolling motion of the fingers. Other signs include masklike facies, slow, monotonous speech, and drooling which are caused by muscle rigidity. The skin is moist and oily. Eyes are dry because of infrequent blinking. Options 1, 3, and 4 are therefore incorrect.
CN: Physiological integrity
CA: Medical/surgical nursing

27. Correct answer - 3. Following head surgery or head injury, clear or yellow drainage from the nose or ears may indicate the leakage of spinal fluid. The presence of glucose in the secretion or drainage indicates that it is spinal fluid and not mucus. It is critical to differentiate between spinal fluid and mucus so that appropriate interventions can be taken in the event that it is spinal fluid. Options 1 and 4: Because leakage of spinal fluid is more serious than producing mucus (as with a cold) these are not the most important question. Option 3: Clear nasal drainage is not an adversee effect of Decadron.
CN: Physiological integrity
CA: Medical/surgical nursing

28. Correct answer - 4. When the child has massive generalized edema, the scrotum is particularly edematous and needs to be supported on a soft pad to relieve tension. Options 1, 2, and 3: The child should be allowed to assume a position of comfort. While the skin is massively edematous, it is very prone to break down. Thus, massage with any type of substance would be too traumatic. There is no need to apply elastic bandages to the child's legs because the edema is not dependent.
CN: Safe, effective care environment
CA: Pediatric nursing

29. Correct answer - 1. Preventing TB involves maintaining an optimum state of health with adequate nutrition and rest. Options 2 and 3: The most common tuberculosis skin test is the tine test, which is administered at about 1 year of age and every several years throughout childhood. Therefore, these two options are incorrect. Option 4: Pyridoxine (vitamin B_6) is used to treat the neuropathy associated with isoniazid (used to treat TB).
CN: Safe, effective care environment
CA: Pediatric nursing

30. Correct answer - 3. A client who has pulmonary edema has respiratory distress. The high-Fowler's position promotes expansion of the client's lungs, which should help to relieve the respiratory distress. Other interventions will also be required to relieve the client's distress, such as diuretics, rapid digitalization, aminophylline I.V., oxygen, etc. Options 1, 2, and 4: Elevating his extremities would increase venous return and make his condition worse. Although he will be attached to a cardiac monitor and have an I.V. infusion, these should be done after positioning him to promote respiratory and cardiac functioning.
CN: Physiological integrity
CA: Medical/surgical nursing

31. Correct answer - 3. Myxedema or hypothyroidism clients are given Synthroid or other thyroid medicine daily for the rest of their lives. Options 1, 2, and 4: She will be sensitive to cold. Surgical intervention is done for hyperthyroidism, not hypothyroidism. Typically, clients with myxedema gain weight because their metabolism is slow. To some extent, weight gain will not be as much of a problem once they get thyroid medication, but even so, they may still gain some weight.
CN: Physiological integrity
CA: Medical/surgical nursing

32. Correct answer - 4. Other symptoms of chronic open-angle glaucoma include loss of peripheral vision, headaches in the brow area, and frequent changes of glasses in persons over age 40. Such symptoms typically develop gradually. Options 1, 2, and 3: Seeing moving spots or floaters is a classic symptom of retinal detachment; and a gradual decrease in visual acuity and loss of

color perception are indicative of other problems (e.g., cataracts).
CN: Physiological integrity
CA: Medical/surgical nursing

33. Correct answer - 4. In the working phase of the relationship, the client is actively involved and assumes responsibility for his healing. Option 1: Requesting information about what to expect, as well as testing limits, are part of the orientation phase of a nurse-client relationship. Option 2: Addressing the nurse by first name is not a characteristic of any particular phase of a therapeutic relationship. Option 3: Expressing sadness about the end of the relationship is typical of the termination phase of a nurse-client relationship.
CN: Psychosocial integrity
CA: Mental health nursing

34. Correct answer - 1. The long incision of a mastectomy can be very unsightly and, therefore, upsetting to the client. She needs to know that, in time, redness, swelling, and irregularity of the incision will decrease, the scar will become less prominent, and tissues will become more normal in color. Option 2: This is not supportive and tells the client how she should feel. Option 3: This does not respond to the client's concern about her appearance. Option 4: This changes the subject from the client's concern about her incision to other people.
CN: Psychosocial integrity
CA: Mental health nursing

35. Correct answer - 4. Staff who practice when they are chemically impaired place clients at risk for harm and the employing agency at risk for liability for negligent actions. Therefore, the nurse's supervisor should be informed about the situation and should help verify perceptions and clarify procedures. Options 1, 2, and 3: Sending the staff member home is not the *best* action initially because the supervisor should first be consulted. More information would need to be obtained before referring the staff member to AA. Harm to clients and the staff member can also

result from non-client care tasks and would tend to maintain denial of the problem.
CN: Safe, effective care environment
CA: Pediatric nursing

36. Correct answer - 1. Liquid iron stains the teeth, so the method of choice is one that best keeps the Feosol from coming in contact with the girl's teeth. Of these choices, the medicine dropper placed well back on her tongue will accomplish that best. Options 2, 3, and 4 would let the liquid to come in contact with her teeth.
CN: Safe, effective care environment
CA: Pediatric nursing

37. Correct answer - 4. Infants with cleft palates are particularly susceptible to middle ear infections because of commensurate eustachian tube inefficiency. Therefore, to avoid middle ear infections and reduce the risk of resultant hearing loss, upper respiratory tract infections need to be treated immediately. Options 1 and 2 are not necessary for these infants. Option 3: Infants such as these are difficult to feed and once a method that works well for the infant and parents is found, it is advisable to stay with it.
CN: Physiological integrity
CA: Pediatric nursing

38. Correct answer - 3. Spastic bladder is caused by a lesion of the spinal cord above the voiding reflex arc, which results in a loss of conscious sensation and cerebral motor control. The bladder empties on reflex. Options 1, 2, and 4 are therefore incorrect.
CN: Physiological integrity
CA: Medical/surgical nursing

39. Correct answer - 2. During a myelogram, the head of the x-ray table is tilted so that the course of the contrast medium in the subarachnoid space can be observed radioscopically. Options 1, 3, and 4: Because the contrast medium is injected into the spine, the groin area does not need to be shaved. Moreover, the client will not be asked to hold his breath. When an oil-based contrast medium has been used, the client should lie in a recumbent

position for several (usually 12 to 24) hours.
CN: Safe, effective care environment
CA: Medical/surgical nursing

40. Correct answer - 1. Forceful nose blowing by a child with a platelet count this low would produce hemorrhage. Options 2, 3, and 4: Vitamin C will have no positive effect in control of the bleeding tendencies associated with a low platelet count. Knowing the urinary pH will not alter therapy for a low platelet count. Although immunizations with live vaccines are generally discontinued for children with ALL, it is not because of the bleeding tendencies but because of the immunosuppression these children experience.
CN: Physiological integrity
CA: Pediatric nursing

41. Correct answer - 1. An apical pulse rate of 90/minute for a child of this age is normal. Lanoxin should not be given to a child of this age if the heart rate is under 70/min. Options 2, 3, and 4: There is no reason to give one-half the dose, to wait and retake the pulse before giving the Lanoxin, or to discuss this situation with the health care provider.
CN: Physiological integrity
CA: Pediatric nursing

42. Correct answer - 3. The client is reporting symptoms suggestive of pregnancy-induced hypertension. Therefore, her urine should be checked for the presence of protein. Options 1, 2, and 4: The height of the fundus, the fetal heart rate, and the presence of human placental lactogen in maternal blood have lower priorities in the assessment of this client.
CN: Health promotion and maintenance
CA: Maternity nursing

43. Correct answer - 3. Rejection is the leading cause of graft failure. Symptoms also include edema, sudden weight gain, hypertension and general malaise. In addition, serum creatinine and blood urea nitrogen values are elevated and proteinuria occurs. Options 1 and 4: Although acute kidney failure and urinary tract obstruction

may exhibit some of the same symptoms as graft rejection, graft rejection should be suspected when these symptoms occur during the first several days after transplant. Option 2: Cystitis is usually manifested by urinary urgency, frequency, and burning and/or pain on urination.
CN: Physiological integrity
CA: Medical/surgical nursing

44. Correct answer - 4. To prevent the spread of infection, clients should be taught how to properly dispose of their secretions. Options 1, 2, and 3: In general, the client can return to work when his symptoms subside and does not have to wait until the medication regimen is completed which may be up to 9 months. Family members have already been exposed to the disease, so disposable eating utensils are unnecessary. The client is considered noninfectious when two successive sputum cultures are negative.
CN: Physiological integrity
CA: Medical/surgical nursing

45. Correct answer - 2. At 20 weeks gestation, the height of the fundus is at the umbilicus. Options 1 and 4: The fundus is at the symphysis pubis at 12 weeks and at the xiphoid at 40 weeks gestation. Option 3: The costal margins are not generally used as landmarks for the uterine fundus.
CN: Health promotion and maintenance
CA: Maternity nursing

46. Correct answer - 2. After birth, the most common problem of an infant of a diabetic mother (IDM) is hypoglycemia. Options 1, 3, and 4: An IDM is at risk for polycythemia, rather than anemia; hypocalcemia, rather than hypercalcemia; and hypophosphatemia, rather than hyperphosphatemia.
CN: Health promotion and maintenance
CA: Maternity nursing

47. Correct answer - 3. After the flames are put out, stopping the burn process is the next important goal. This can be done by placing cool water on the burn area, by immersing the burned part in water, or by placing cool compresses on the burn

area. Options 1, 2, and 4: These are incorrect.
CN: Physiological integrity
CA: Pediatric nursing

48. Correct answer - 4. The client is experiencing an alteration in information processing (delusions) that makes effectively filtering incoming stimuli difficult. Therefore, focusing the client on one reality-based activity at a time, using clear, concise instructions, is helpful. Options 1, 2, and 3: The delusions should not be reinforced by dwelling on them, nor should they be directly challenged. Rational explanations will only make the client adhere more firmly to her delusion.
CN: Psychosocial integrity
CA: Mental health nursing

49. Correct answer - 3. When the client is unable to take care of her own hygiene needs (because of low self-esteem and psychomotor retardation), the nurse should help or, if necessary, do the activities for the client. Option 1: Rather than *telling* the client that she cares, the nurse should *show* her that she cares by attending to her care needs. Option 2: The depressed client should not be given the option to refuse participation in activities of daily living or expected unit activities. Option 4: Although remaining silently with the client may convey concern, getting her mobilized is more important.
CN: Psychosocial integrity
CA: Mental health nursing

50. Correct answer - 1. Addisonian crisis may be caused by stress (e.g., from infection, surgery, trauma, hemorrhage, or psychological distress) or sudden withdrawal of adrenocortical hormone replacement therapy. Of the choices given, having the flu, an infection, is the most likely precipitating factor. Options 2, 3, and 4: Clients who have Addison's disease may be taught to increase their salt intake in hot and humid weather when they are apt to perspire and to increase the dose of glucocorticoids during periods of stress. Doses are usually doubled when minor stress occurs and tripled when major stress occurs. The onset of menstruation, which may or may not be stressful to the client, is not as clear a precipitating factor as

the infection (flu).
CN: Physiological integrity
CA: Medical/surgical nursing

51. Correct answer - 4. The normal range for a blood urea nitrogen (BUN) test is 8 to 25 mg/dl. Because the client's result is elevated, the health care provider should be notified. Options 1, 2, and 3 are incorrect. The results all fall within the normal ranges for their respective tests.
CN: Safe, effective care environment
CA: Medical/surgical nursing

52. Correct answer - 4. Prophylactic chest physical therapy needs to be done at least twice a day to help prevent respiratory infections. Often adolescents rebel and neglect their self-care routines. So when caring for an adolescent who has CF and a respiratory infection, the nurse must determine if lack of prophylactic chest physical therapy is contributing to the infection. Options 1, 2, and 3: None of them have anything to do with the predisposing factors of a respiratory infection in the adolescent with CF.
CN: Physiological integrity
CA: Pediatric nursing

53. Correct answer - 3. Passive arm exercises usually are started on the evening of surgery to prevent shoulder stiffness, which can lead to frozen shoulder. Options 1, 2, and 4: Osteoarthritis is a noninflammatory degenerative joint disease; synovitis is the inflammation of a synovial membrane; and tendonitis is an inflammation of tendons and of tendon muscle attachments.
CN: Physiological integrity
CA: Medical/surgical nursing

54. Correct answer - 2. In acute pulmonary edema, blood serum is rapidly effused into the pulmonary interstitial tissues and alveoli. This, in turn, interferes with the oxygenation of blood and results in poor tissue perfusion. Thus, altered tissue perfusion should get priority in the client's care. Option 1, 3, and 4: Although all of them may be important in the client's care, they are not as important as altered tissue perfusion.

CN: Physiological integrity
CA: Medical/surgical nursing

55. Correct answer - 2. Exposing the nipples to air and sunlight will help toughen them. Options 1 and 4: Soap and antiseptics should not be used on the nipples because they remove protective oils that keep nipples supple. Option 3: Plastic bra liners are not recommended because they retain moisture against the nipples.
CN: Health promotion and maintenance
CA: Maternity nursing

56. Correct answer - 4. The infant has experienced cold stress and is being rewarmed. Rapid warming may cause apneic spells and acidosis in an infant. Option 1: Newborns do not shiver. Option 2: Acrocyanosis of the hands and feet is normally found in the newborn. Option 3: Assessment of the fontanels is not the first priority for this newborn.
CN: Health promotion and maintenance
CA: Maternity nursing

57. Correct answer - 1. Women who practice pica may eat relatively large amounts of substances, such as laundry starch or clay. Such ingestions interfere with good nutrition and are associated with iron-deficiency anemia. Options 2, 3, and 4 are not associated with pica.
CN: Health promotion and maintenance
CA: Maternity nursing

58. Correct answer - 1. Among the danger signals for adolescent suicide are symptoms of depression and the inability to communicate with parents. Other symptoms include neglect of personal appearance (the opposite of option 2), no close friends (the opposite of option 3), and lack of involvement in any school activities (the opposite of option 4).
CN: Psychosocial integrity
CA: Mental health nursing

59. Correct answer - 4. Judgment is assessed by asking the client to evaluate a hypothetical situation and make a decision about a course of action.

Option 1: Calculating relationships about currencies of different sizes tests arithmetic ability and general intellectual functioning. Option 2: Identifying similarities tests abstract thinking. Option 3: Interpreting proverbs tests abstract thinking and the ability to conceptualize.
CN: Psychosocial integrity
CA: Mental health nursing

60. Correct answer - 2. In the acute phase of laryngotracheobronchitis, children are quite ill. In addition to severe respiratory symptoms (e.g., dyspnea, laryngeal spasm, cough, cyanosis), they may have an elevated temperature, cold, clammy skin, and a rapid pulse. Planning ways to conserve the child's energy is particularly important. Once the acute phase has passed, more attention can be given to the other goals. Options 1, 3, and 4 are therefore incorrect.
CN: Physiological integrity
CA: Pediatric nursing

61. Correct answer - 3. In TB, multiple drug regimens are used to destroy as many tubercle bacilli as quickly as possible and to minimize the development of resistant tubercle bacilli. Although the tubercle bacillus is susceptible to several drugs, it can develop resistance to all of them. Options 1, 2, and 4 are therefore incorrect.
CN: Physiological integrity
CA: Medical/surgical nursing

62. Correct answer - 4. With inactivated antigens, such as DTP, adverse effects are most likely to occur within a few hours or days of administration and usually are limited to local tenderness, erythema, and swelling at the injection site, low grade fever, and behavior changes. Options 1, 2, and 3 are incorrect.
CN: Physiological integrity
CA: Pediatric nursing

63. Correct answer - 3. The client is at risk for violence to others because he is experiencing command hallucinations. The safety of the other clients and staff must be assured; therefore, the diagnosis given in option 3 has a higher priority than options 1, 2, or 4.

CN: Psychosocial integrity
CA: Mental health nursing

64. Correct answer - 3. To help an elderly person sleep, a bedtime ritual should be encouraged. Option 1: Bedtime sedation may help a person get to sleep, but sedatives change the normal sleep pattern, which may make the client wake up more during the night or feel drowsy and lethargic the next day. Option 2: The time it takes to fall asleep is related to the length of time from the last sleep period; therefore, elders may find that they can fall asleep at night if they nap in the morning rather than taking an afternoon nap. Option 4: Exercise and activity during the day should be encouraged, not discouraged, because they increase the likelihood of falling asleep at night.
CN: Physiological integrity
CA: Mental health nursing

65. Correct answer - 4. Classic symptoms of pyloric stenosis include projectile vomiting, hunger, irritability, failure to gain (or even lose) weight, a palpable olive-shaped tumor in the epigastrium just to the right of the umbilicus, visible gastric peristaltic waves that move from left to right across the epigastrium, and those symptoms associated with dehydration (e.g., decreased elasticity of the skin, sunken eyeballs, and loss of subcutaneous tissue). Option 1, 2, and 3 are therefore incorrect.
CN: Physiological integrity
CA: Pediatric nursing

66. Correct answer - 3. With profound liver failure, ammonia and other toxic substances accumulate in the blood because the damaged liver cells fail to detoxify and convert to urea the ammonia that is constantly entering the bloodstream as a result of its absorption from the gastrointestinal tract and its liberation from kidney and muscle cells. The increased ammonia in the blood can result in hepatic encephalopathy or coma. Circumstances that increase blood ammonia content tend to aggravate or precipitate hepatic coma. Mycifradin is given to inhibit nitrogen-forming bacteria, which are capable of converting urea to ammonia, in the gastrointestinal tract.

Options 1, 2, and 4: Creatinine is elevated in nephritis and chronic renal disease; an elevated acid phosphatase is seen in prostate cancer, hyperparathyroidism, and Paget's disease; and haptoglobin is elevated in pregnancy, estrogen therapy, and chronic infections and inflammations.
CN: Physiological integrity
CA: Medical/surgical nursing

67. Correct answer - 2. The client should be observed for elevation of all vital signs, including elevated blood pressure and hyperthermia rather than hypothermia (option 4). Option 1: Hypoglycemia, not hyperglycemia may occur during withdrawal because alcohol depletes the glycogen stored in the liver. Option 3: Hypouricemia is not associated with withdrawal from alcohol.
CN: Psychosocial integrity
CA: Mental health nursing

68. Correct answer - 2. In acute or chronic renal failure, hyperphosphatemia develops because of the altered ability of the kidneys to excrete phosphates. To reduce serum phosphate levels, clients are given phosphate-binding agents or gels (like Amphojel) and advised to limit dietary phosphates. Options 1, 3, and 4: Amphojel *is not* given for any of these purposes.
CN: Safe, effective care environment
CA: Medical/surgical nursing

69. Correct answer - 3. The partial thromboplastin time (PTT) is used to monitor a client's response to heparin sodium. The goal is to achieve a PTT of 1½ to 2½ times the control or normal level. Options 1, 2, and 4: The results of a prothrombin time (options 1 and 2) are used to monitor a client's response to Coumadin. The values given in option 4 are too high, which would put the client at risk for bleeding.
CN: Physiological integrity
CA: Medical/surgical nursing

70. Correct answer - 3. Following a bronchoscopy, the client should be monitored for symptoms of laryngeal edema and laryngospasms

which include stridor or dyspnea. Options 1, 2, and 4: None of them are associated with complications of a bronchoscopy. It is not unusual for a client's sputum to be slightly blood-tinged after the procedure.
CN: Safe, effective care environment
CA: Medical/surgical nursing

71. Correct answer - 1. The child with a hip dysplasia exhibits signs of shortening of the femur on the affected side. The thigh or gluteal folds are increased and abduction of the affected side is limited. With corrective surgery, these should disappear. Options 2, 3, and 4 are incorrect.
CN: Safe, effective care environment
CA: Pediatric nursing

72. Correct answer - 1. A client who is taking large doses of Lasix or who is taking Lasix and an antihypertensive at the same time is at risk of developing postural or orthostatic hypotension. Thus, he should be instructed to rise slowly from a lying or sitting position. Options 2, 3, and 4: There is no need the client include any of these activities in his care.
CN: Physiological integrity
CA: Medical/surgical nursing

73. Correct answer - 2. Following most prostatectomies, the client usually dribbles urine, which may continue for 6 to 12 months. Options 1, 3, and 4: Because it takes the prostatic fossa 6 to 8 weeks to heal, strenuous activities such as long automobile rides and sexual intercourse should be avoided as they may cause bleeding. The client should void as soon as the desire is felt.
CN: Safe, effective care environment
CA: Medical/surgical nursing

74. Correct answer - 4. One of the contraindications to atropine sulfate is open-angle glaucoma because it can increase intraocular pressure in these clients. Therefore, the nurse should contact the health care provider who wrote the order to remind him that the client has glaucoma. Options 1, 2, and 3: Clients who are to have an abdominal hysterectomy do have an abdominal prep and shave and may or may not have a vaginal douche with tap water or Betadine. There is nothing atypical about the Demerol order.
CN: Safe, effective care environment
CA: Medical/surgical nursing

75. Correct answer - 4. When a nasogastric tube is inserted, the client does not need to cough. Therefore, this statement by the student needs to be clarified and corrected. Options 1, 2, and 3 are all correct and thus do not need to be clarified.
CN: Safe, effective care environment
CA: Medical/surgical nursing

76. Correct answer - 4. The client's symptoms indicate that he is in diabetic ketoacidosis. Therefore, the nurse should question administering 50% dextrose in water (which may be given if the client has severe hypoglycemia). Options 1, 2, and 3: With diabetic ketoacidosis, the three main goals of care are to correct dehydration, electrolyte loss, and acidosis. To do this, 0.9% normal saline is administered at a high rate, up to 40 mEq/hour of potassium chloride is given I.V., and Regular insulin is infused at a slow continuous rate.
CN: Safe, effective care environment
CA: Medical/surgical nursing

77. Correct answer - 4. A depressed client may conceal medication in his cheek in order to accumulate enough medication to overdose. Options 1, 2 and 3: The precautions about food, activity, and weight gain are not relevant to the client's plan of care.
CN: Psychosocial integrity
CA: Mental health nursing

78. Correct answer - 3. The duration of a contraction is timed from the beginning of the contraction to the end of that contraction. Option 1: Describes timing of the frequency of contractions. Option 4: Describes the period of relaxation between contractions. Option 2 is not a measurement generally made and does not reflect the duration of a contraction.
CN: Health promotion and maintenance
CA: Maternity nursing

79. Correct answer - 4. Methadone is a synthetic narcotic that does not produce the high that is associated with heroin. Option 1 and 2: Methadone is addictive and can be given subcutaneously and intramuscularly, as well as orally. Option 3: Withdrawal from methadone is accompanied by physical symptoms that are less intense but more prolonged than the symptoms experienced in heroin withdrawal.
CN: Physiological integrity
CA: Mental health nursing

80. Correct answer - 2. Following a supratentorial craniotomy, the client is maintained with the head of the bed elevated 30 to 45 degrees, and not flat. Options 1, 3, and 4: Clients with supratentorial craniotomies are at risk for seizures, so padding the side rails is appropriate. There is no reason to suspect that the client should not be receiving oxygen and at that rate. Clients with craniotomies can be positioned on either side or the back. If a large tumor has been removed, however, avoid placing the client on the operative side.
CN: Safe, effective care environment
CA: Medical/surgical nursing

81. Correct answer - 1. Risk factors for essential hypertension include advancing age, male, Afro-American race, family history of hypertension, obesity, smoking, excessive alcohol intake, high-sodium diet, emotional stress, and atherosclerosis. Options 2, 3, and 4 are not risk factors for essential hypertension.
CN: Safe, effective care environment
CA: Medical/surgical nursing

82. Correct answer - 1. An exercise electrocardiograph (ECG) helps determine the heart's functional capacity and to screen for asymptomatic coronary artery disease by assessing the cardiovascular response to an increased workload. During the test, the client is attached to an ECG machine and performs an exercise (i.e., riding a stationary bicycle or walking on a treadmill). The client's blood pressure and ECG are closely monitored during the test. Options 2 and 3 are incorrect although they all partially

describe other tests. Option 2 partially describes the purpose of phonocardiography; option 3, echocardiography. Option 4 describes some of the purposes of hemodynamic monitoring.
CN: Safe, effective care environment
CA: Medical/surgical nursing

83. Correct answer - 2. Recommended age of MMR immunizations is 15 months. Options 1, 3, and 4 therefore are incorrect.
CN: Health promotion and maintenance
CA: Pediatric nursing

84. Correct answer - 2. The primary factor--and the one that is responsible for the multiple clinical manifestations of CF--is mechanical obstruction caused by increased viscosity of mucous gland secretions. Small passages in organs such as the pancreas and bronchioles become obstructed as secretions precipitate and coagulate to form concretions in glands and ducts. Option 4: In CF, the oxygen-carbon dioxide exchange is reduced. Option 1 and 3: Allergies and/or inflammation are not *causes* of the respiratory symptoms demonstrated in cystic fibrosis; if they exist, they are a *result* of the disease.
CN: Physiological integrity
CA: Pediatric nursing

85. Correct answer - 1. In Kegel's exercises, the pubococcygeal muscle is alternately tightened and relaxed. Option 2: A pelvic tilt exercise is described in this option. Option 3: This describes Hoffman's exercises, used to increase nipple protractility. Option 4: This describes the "tailor sit," used to stretch the muscles of the inner thighs.
CN: Health promotion and maintenance
CA: Maternity nursing

86. Correct answer - 1. Dilantin has many adverse effects. In addition to gingival hyperplasia, others include dizziness, drowsiness, hypotension, nausea, vomiting, loss of taste, weight loss, agranulocytosis, and hyperglycemia. Therefore, options 2, 3, and 4 are incorrect.
CN: Physiological integrity
CA: Medical/surgical nursing

87. Correct answer - 2. Because a needle is placed in the spinal column, children (adults also) need to remain still and immobile to prevent trauma or injury to the spinal column. Options 1, 3, and 4: There is no need to restrict fluids before this test; only a small Band-aid is required for the puncture site; and there is no need to check urine specific gravity.
CN: Safe, effective care environment
CA: Pediatric nursing

88. Correct answer - 1. Thyroid crisis or thyroid storm is caused by a sudden increase in the secretion of thyroxine or by inadequate suppression of thyroid activity preoperatively. In thyroid storm, all of the body processes are speeded up which results in markedly elevated vital signs. Options 2, 3, and 4: These vital signs are within normal ranges for a client who has had a thyroidectomy.
CN: Physiological integrity
CA: Medical/surgical nursing

89. Correct answer - 2. Following oral administration, sucralfate and gastric acid react to form a viscous, adhesive paste-like substance that is resistant to further action with an acid. This paste adheres to the gastric mucosa, protecting the damaged mucosa against further destruction from ulcerogenic secretions and drugs. Options 1, 3, and 4 are therefore incorrect. Sucralfate *inhibits* the secretion of pepsin.
CN: Physiological integrity
CA: Medical/surgical nursing

90. Correct answer - 2. This comment suggests dehiscence (partial separation) or evisceration (complete separation) of the client's wound. Thus, the nurse should assess the wound immediately. Options 1, 3, and 4 all indicate the return of peristalsis and may indicate that the peritonitis is subsiding.
CN: Physiological integrity
CA: Medical/surgical nursing

PERSONAL DIAGNOSTIC PROFILE
(see the following page for instructions)

QUESTION NUMBER																						Totals

TEST-TAKING SKILLS

Misread the question																						
Missed important point																						
Forgot fact or concept																						
Applied wrong fact or concept																						
Drew wrong conclusion																						
Incorrectly evaluated distractors																						
Mistakenly selected answer choice																						
Read into the question																						
Made a wrong guess																						
Misunderstood question																						

CLIENT NEED CATEGORIES

Safe, effective care environment																						
Physiological integrity																						
Psychosocial integrity																						
Health promotion and maintenance																						

CLINICAL AREAS

Pediatric nursing																						
Maternity nursing																						
Medical/surgical nursing																						
Mental health nursing																						

HOW TO SCORE AND USE THE DIAGNOSTIC PROFILE

In the top "QUESTION NUMBER" row of boxes, mark each question number you answered wrong. Under each question number, check the box in the "TEST TAKING SKILLS" section that is the most appropriate reason you answered the question incorrectly. Do the same for the "CLIENT NEED CATEGORIES" AND "CLINICAL AREAS" section. The client need and clinical area codes follow the rationale. Total the number of check marks, by line, in the "Totals" column. This provides you with a profile of your weak areas that should be improve upon prior to taking the NCLEX-RN.

CALCULATION OF SUBSCORES

After you score your test, determine your subscores in these areas by filling in the following two grids.

CLINICAL AREA

	Medical/surgical nursing	Pediatric nursing	Maternity nursing	Mental health nursing
Number of questions	40	23	11	16
Number incorrect				
Number correct				
Percent correct*				

*To determine the percent correct, divide the number of items answered correctly by the total number of items and multiply the results by 100.

CLIENT NEED

	Safe, effective care environment	Physiological integrity	Psychosocial integrity	Health promotion & maintenance
Number of questions	26	41	11	12
Number incorrect				
Number correct				
Percent correct*				

*To determine the percent correct in each category, divide the number of items answered correctly by the total number of items and multiply the result by 100.

Note: This is a short test with a limited sample of items in each category. Therefore, if a score in any category is less than 75% correct, further study is strongly advised.

Common abbreviations

AA	Alcoholics Anonymous
ABGs	arterial blood gases
ACE	angiotensin converting enzyme
ADA	American Dietetic Association
ADL	activities of daily living
AF	atrial fibrillation
AHA	American Heart Association
AIDS	acquired immunodeficiency syndrome
ANA	American Nurses Association
BCE	breast clinical examination
b.i.d.	twice daily
bpm	beats per minute
BMR	basal metabolic rate
BSA	body surface area
BSE	breast self-examination
BUN	blood urea nitrogen
BZD	benzodiazepines
CA	Cocaine Anonymous
CAL	chronic airflow limitation
CBC	complete blood count
CDC	Centers for Disease Control and Prevention
CF	cystic fibrosis
CHD	congenital hip dysplasia
CK	creatine kinase
CL	cleft lip
CNS	central nervous system
COPD	chronic obstructive pulmonary disease
CP	cleft palate
CPD	cephalopelvic disproportion
CPR	cardiopulmonary resuscitation
CPT	chest physical therapy
CSF	cerebral spinal fluid
CT	computed tomography
CVA	cerebral vascular accident
CVP	central venous pressure

DDH	developmental dysplasia of the hip
DM	diabetes mellitus
DOT	directly observed therapy
DT	delirium tremens
DTP	diphtheria, tetanus, pertussis
DVT	deep vein thrombosis
EA	esophageal atresia
ECG	electrocardiogram
ELISA	enzyme-linked immunosorbent assay
ESR	erythrocyte sedimentation rate
FHT	fetal heart tones
GAD	generalized anxiety disorder
GDM	gestational diabetes mellitus
GERD	gastroesophageal reflux disease
GI	gastrointestinal
GTT	glucose tolerance test
HBA_{1c}	glycosylated hemoglobin
HBV	hepatitis B vaccine
hCG	human chorionic gonadotropin
HDL	high-density lipoproteins
Hgb	hemoglobin
Hib	Haemophilus influenza type b (vaccine)
HIV	human immunodeficiency virus
HMO	health maintenance organization
HOB	head of bed
hPL	human placental lactogen
ICP	intracranial pressure
IDA	iron-deficiency anemia
IICP	increased intracranial pressure
I.M.	intramuscular
INR	international normalized ratio
I&O	intake and output
IS	incentive spirometry
I.V.	intravenous
IVP	intravenous pyelogram

LDH	lactic dehydrogenase
LDL	low-density lipoproteins
LGA	large for gestational age
LOC	level of consciousness
L:S	lecithin synthesis

MAOI	monamine oxidase inhibitor
MAP	mean arterial pressure
$MgSO_4$	magnesium sulfate
MI	myocardial infarction
MMR	measles, mumps, rubella (vaccine)
MRI	magnetic resonance imaging

NA	Narcotics Anonymous
NCSBN	National Council of State Boards of Nursing
NG	nasogastric
NPO	non per os (nothing by mouth)
NSAID	non-steroidal antiinflammatory drug
NSS	normal saline solution
NST	non-stress test

O/CD	obsessive-compulsive disorder
OCT	oxytocin challenge test
OM	otitis media
OPV	oral poliovirus (vaccine)
OTC	over-the-counter

PCA	patient-controlled analgesia
PE	pulmonary embolus
PEEP	positive end-expiratory pressure
PIH	pregnancy-induced hypertension
PO	per os (by mouth)
PPD	purified protein derivative
PPOs	preferred provider organizations
prn	pro re nata (as necessary)
PSA	prostate-specific antigen
PT	prothrombin time
PTSD	posttraumatic stress disorder
PTT	partial thromboplastin time
PVC	premature ventricular contraction
PVR	pulmonary vascular resistance

q.d.	every day
q.i.d.	four times daily

RA	rheumatoid arthritis
RAD	reactive airway disease
RBC	red blood cells
ROM	rupture of membranes
RSV	respiratory syncytial virus

SAD	seasonal affective disorder
SC	subcutaneously
SGA	small for gestational age
SNS	sympathetic nervous system
SP	suicide precautions

TB	tuberculosis
TCA	tricyclics
Td	tetanus and diphtheria (vaccine)
TEF	tracheoesophageal fistule
TH	thyroid hormone
t.i.d.	three times daily
TOF	tetralogy of Fallot
TPN	total parenteral nutrition

UAP	unlicensed assistive personnel
URI	upper respiratory infection
UTI	urinary tract infection

VSD	ventricular septal defect

WBC	white blood cells
WNL	within normal limits